Quiet Triumphs

Harnessing the Power of Introversion

by

Dr. ant

Quiet Triumphs: Harnessing the Power of Introversion

Contents

Introduction

In a world that often seems to idolize the gregarious achievements of extroverts, introverts have quietly carved their path, contributing profoundly to the tapestry of society. As more individuals begin to understand the unique strengths that introversion offers, there's a noticeable shift in how both introverts and extroverts view this personality trait. This book is dedicated to empowering introverts while reshaping societal perspectives, offering insights, strategies, and validation for those who resonate with the introverted spectrum.

Introversion, often misunderstood and undervalued, holds immense potential. It's not simply about shyness or reclusiveness; rather, it encompasses a rich world of introspection, creativity, and profound thought. Many introverts thrive in environments that allow for solitude and deep reflection. This inner world can be a reservoir of ideas and insights that, when tapped into, can lead to groundbreaking innovations and empathetic leadership.

The journey to recognizing and celebrating introversion begins with understanding. Society frequently overlooks the quieter virtues of introverts, sometimes perceiving them as aloof or disengaged. Yet it's these very qualities that empower introverts to notice subtleties others might miss and to develop insights into complex problems. The strengths of introverts are diverse, stretching across fields from science to the arts, proving their valuable contributions.

As societal norms begin to shift, there's a growing recognition of the strengths inherent in introversion. The clichéd idea of the gregarious leader is gradually giving way to understanding that success can equally stem from an introverted approach. Leaders who listen more than they speak, who ponder before they decide, who lead with quiet confidence rather than brash declarations, have had an undeniable impact throughout history.

At the heart of this discussion is a crucial paradigm shift in how people perceive productivity and success. It's easy to assume that productivity is synonymous with constant interaction and action, yet many introverts demonstrate that effective leadership and success come through thoughtful planning, strategic decision-making, and the ability to connect deeply with others on a more personal level. These qualities bring balance and depth to teams and organizations.

Recognizing one's introverted nature and learning to embrace it as a strength rather than a weakness is a transformative process. The journey involves overcoming societal biases that favor extroversion, thereby fostering a greater sense of self-acceptance. Building confidence from within, understanding one's preferences, and leveraging them for personal and professional growth can create a fulfilling and impactful life.

While navigating social and professional landscapes, introverts often face challenges that require unique approaches. Whether it's choosing a career path, engaging in effective communication, or participating in social events, introverts can employ tailored strategies to succeed without compromising their natural tendencies. This book will explore these strategies to empower introverts in making authentic choices that align with their inner selves.

By thriving in solitude and using it as a time for creativity, introverts can unlock sources of inspiration that fuel their passions and projects. Introverts often find immense joy in cultivating deep connections, albeit fewer, rather than spreading themselves thin across numerous superficial interactions. This quality can lead to more meaningful and lasting personal and professional relationships.

Introverts today face unique opportunities and challenges, especially with the rapid advances in technology and the evolving social landscape. Embracing these changes with an introverted lens can provide them with tools and platforms to showcase their strengths uniquely. Technology offers introverts the spaces to engage on their terms, allowing them to thrive and contribute significantly to the digital age.

As society marches forward, there's an exciting opportunity for introverts to redefine what success looks like, on their own terms. There's a power in blending the quietness of introversion with the extroverted demands of modern life, crafting a life that is both fulfilling and successful. Each chapter that follows seeks to delve deeper into these themes, guided by stories, research, and practical advice designed to uplift and support introverts as they embark on their personal and collective journeys.

Ultimately, this book aspires to inspire introverts to not only accept their nature but to harness it as a source of strength. By shifting societal narratives and offering a renewed perspective on introversion, we hope to foster inclusivity and understanding, promoting a world where introverts and extroverts can appreciate and balance each other's unique gifts.

Chapter 1: Understanding Introversion

Introversion isn't just about shyness or preferring solitude; it's a unique way of processing the world that can be deeply enriching. For those with an introverted disposition, understanding this trait can lead to immense personal growth and empowerment. Unlike extroverts who thrive on external stimuli, introverts draw energy from within, finding richness in reflection and depth in solitude. This internal orientation involves a distinct neurological wiring, making introverts adept at introspection and innovative problem-solving. Recognizing and valuing these qualities can unlock potential that goes unnoticed in a society that often celebrates outgoing personalities. Embracing introversion means harnessing quiet power, not just for personal fulfillment but also for contributing profound insights in professional settings. By understanding the biological and psychological roots of introversion, introverts and extroverts alike can learn to appreciate the diverse strengths this influential trait brings to the table.

Defining Introversion and Extroversion

To truly understand introversion, we must start by defining what sets it apart from extroversion. These terms are more than just labels; they describe essential aspects of personality. While introversion and extroversion are often viewed as opposites, they're actually different points on a spectrum of how individuals respond to external stimuli and recharge their energies. Introverts tend to feel invigorated by solitary reflection and minimal stimulation. Extroverts, on the other hand, draw their energy from social interactions and external engagements. These divergent preferences shape not only our social behaviors but also how we process information, make decisions, and reflect on our experiences.

The notion of introversion and extroversion wasn't coined until early in the 20th century. Carl Jung first brought these terms into the mainstream psychological community, providing a framework that helps people gain insights into their personal approaches to the world. For introverts, stillness and solitude are not just preferences—they're needs that feed their internal thought processes and emotional balance. Extroverts thrive in dynamic environments, engaging with a wide circle of acquaintances and participating in bustling activities to keep their spirits high. Understanding this fundamental distinction can empower introverts to embrace who they are, rather than feeling pressured to conform to societal extroversion ideals.

Let's dive a bit deeper. Contrary to some mainstream perceptions, introversion isn't about shyness or social anxiety. Plenty of introverts enjoy social activities and can engage meaningfully with others; they just often prefer smaller gatherings and require time alone afterward to recharge. Extroverts, in contrast, can gain energy from crowds and dynamic surroundings, seeing solitude not as a refuge but as a desert of experience. This difference is crucial in personal development—acknowledging one's position on the introversion-extroversion spectrum leads to a better understanding of personal strengths and needs.

Modern psychological theories also suggest that these preferences might have both a biological and environmental basis. Some research indicates that introverts experience greater stimulation from novelty and social engagement, which can lead to feeling overwhelmed more quickly than extroverts. Brain activity studies highlight different pathways and responses to dopamine, a neurotransmitter associated with pleasure and reward, suggesting that introverts and extroverts might process external rewards differently. This isn't just science for the sake of curiosity; it offers validation and encouragement to embrace one's natural inclinations.

Beyond these foundational genetics, society and upbringing play significant roles in shaping whether one identifies as introverted or extroverted. Family dynamics, cultural expectations, and educational environments can either nurture or challenge an individual's natural inclinations. For instance, an introverted child in an extroverted family may feel out of place or misunderstood, highlighting the importance of building an awareness and societal narrative that values both introverts and extroverts equally. Our ultimate goal is not to advocate one over the other but to respect and nurture both as valuable parts of the human experience.

Consider the workplace—a traditional arena of extrovert-aligned expectations, where open floor plans, group brainstorming sessions, and constant meetings are more common than ever. Here, introversion and extroversion can sometimes clash, especially if the quiet contributions of introverts are overshadowed by louder, more extroverted voices. Recognizing and valuing diverse input styles ensures everyone can contribute their best. Introverts might shine in solitary, focused projects, or in smaller, more intimate settings where deep connections foster innovation and thoughtful problem-solving. Conversely, extroverts bring energetic networking skills to the table, thriving on collaborative efforts that can drive projects forward swiftly.

In romantic relationships, this balance of introversion and extroversion can either complement or compete, depending on mutual understanding and respect for each partner's needs. Introverts may favor time spent one-on-one, cherishing the depth and quality of interaction, while extroverts might thrive with a larger social circle and the vibrancy of multiple friends and acquaintances. Successful relationships often come down to recognizing these different preferences and finding a harmonious dance between the two ends of the spectrum.

It's all about self-awareness. Introversion and extroversion provide a lens through which individuals can view themselves and others more compassionately. By understanding these dimensions, we not only empower introverts to find their unique strengths but also equip extroverts to appreciate the quiet power of introspection. As we move forward, exploring the biological and psychological bases of these traits, the varied ways introversion manifests will become clearer, leading to a richer understanding of how both introverts and extroverts contribute to a vibrant, balanced society.

The Biological and Psychological Basis of Introversion

Understanding the biology and psychology of introversion is key to demystifying what it means to be an introvert. At its core, introversion isn't just a preference for quiet environments over the bustling chaos of crowds; it's a deeply ingrained attribute shaped both by the brain and by psychological factors. Science reveals that introverts process the world differently than extroverts, offering a unique lens through which to view life's complexities.

Biologically speaking, the foundation of introversion can be traced back to fundamental differences in the brain's wiring. Studies have shown that introverts may have a unique pattern of neuronal activity. For instance, the neural pathways involved in the reward systems of the brain don't work the same way for introverts as they do for extroverts. This alteration results in introverts reacting to external stimuli distinctly, often leading to a preference for internal reflection over external engagement.

One of the significant biological findings relates to the neurotransmitter dopamine. It plays a pivotal role in how we experience rewards, motivation, and pleasure. Introverts tend to be more sensitive to dopamine levels, which means that their threshold for stimulation is lower than that of their extroverted peers. In simple terms, what might energize an extrovert could easily overwhelm an introvert. Due to this sensitivity, introverts often require less external reward to feel content, aligning them more with activities that involve lower stimulus environments.

Beyond dopamine, the reticular activating system (RAS) in the brain also contributes to the introverted experience. The RAS is responsible for regulating sleep and arousal, acting as a gateway through which all information must pass before it's processed by the brain's cortex. Introverts have an RAS that is more easily stimulated, leading to quick exhaustion in high-stimulation environments. This is why parties and crowded meetings can leave introverts feeling drained, while solitude feels rejuvenating.

From a psychological standpoint, introversion ties closely to the way individuals process information. Introverts are often seen as deep thinkers, and this cognitive trait is backed by psychological research. They tend to favor focus over multitasking, diving deeply into subjects of interest. This depth-oriented approach not only enhances their attention to detail but also allows introverts to experience a richer internal dialogue. Creativity, too, often thrives in this deep thought process, enabling introverts to cultivate original ideas and innovative solutions.

Further psychological aspects of introversion include the concept of energy levels. Introverts recharge through solitary activities and intimate settings. This need for solitude isn't a sign of anti-social behavior but a psychological necessity. By understanding and respecting this need, introverts can navigate both personal and professional landscapes while maintaining energy balance and mental well-being.

While these biological and psychological traits paint a picture of introversion, it's important to remember that traits exist on a spectrum. Some individuals might display a blend of both introverted and extroverted characteristics, often referred to as ambiverts. It underscores the understanding that introversion isn't a rigid box, but a fluid space influenced by both innate qualities and external experiences.

Embracing the science behind introversion can lead to greater self-awareness among introverts. Recognizing the unique ways in which their brains function allows introverts to harness their natural strengths effectively. It can shift the focus from trying to "fit in" to a more empowering acknowledgment of the introverted experience. This awareness fosters an environment where introverts can truly thrive, leveraging their disposition to navigate the world on their terms.

As society gradually becomes more aware of these nuances, it becomes essential to celebrate the introverted way of being. By understanding the biological and psychological foundation of introversion, we not only validate the experiences of introverts but also challenge the extro-centric narrative that prevails in many cultures. As new findings unfold, they offer a roadmap for introverts and those seeking to support them, paving the way for environments that cherish and incorporate the quiet power of introversion.

Chapter 2: Embracing the Quiet Power

Introversion often comes with a unique set of strengths that shine brightly once embraced, many of which are frequently overlooked in a society that champions extroverted ideals. By tuning into the quiet power within, introverts can discover an untapped reserve of potential, such as an acute ability to listen with depth, a preference for meaningful connections, and a knack for thoughtful problem-solving. Introverts' tendency to reflect before acting can lead to more deliberate and impactful choices, both personally and professionally. While myths suggest introverts may lack enthusiasm or assertiveness, these misconceptions underestimate the profound ways they contribute to the world. By redefining how we view nearly effortless charisma as the sole marker of strength, we unravel a deeper appreciation for the calm confidence that introverts inherently carry. Celebrating this quiet power not only enriches introverts' own lives but also prompts a cultural shift, moving towards a world that values introspection and deep thought just as much as outgoing expressiveness.

The Strengths of Introverts: An Overview

In a world that often rewards the outspoken and the bold, the quiet strengths of introverts might sometimes be overlooked. Yet, embracing these qualities can be transformative, not just for introverts themselves, but for the society that surrounds them. To truly flourish, introverts need to celebrate and harness their unique capabilities, which are as varied as they are profound.

One of the most remarkable strengths introverts possess is their ability to focus deeply. Unlike extroverts, who may thrive on the buzz of activity, introverts often find their power in sustained concentration. This ability allows them to immerse themselves in tasks, uncovering insights that may elude those who are less able to focus for extended periods. Whether it's solving complex problems or mastering a skill, introverts often find success through deliberate and thoughtful engagement.

Introverts also bring a rich landscape of reflection and introspection. This reflective nature isn't simply about navel-gazing; it is the ability to learn from past experiences and anticipate future challenges. Through introspection, introverts develop a keen sense of self-awareness and emotional intelligence, qualities that contribute to personal growth and the ability to navigate social environments thoughtfully.

Moreover, introverts are often exceptional listeners. In conversations, they are inclined to absorb and reflect upon what others are saying rather than rush in with their viewpoint. This patience and attentiveness can foster deeper, more meaningful connections, as those around them feel truly heard and understood. In both personal interactions and professional environments, this ability to listen actively can build trust and facilitate collaboration.

This deep listening ties into another strength: the capacity for empathy. Introverts, through their reflective and contemplative nature, often exhibit a remarkable ability to understand and empathize with others. They value genuine connections and are adept at tuning into the emotions and perspectives of those around them. This empathetic approach can enrich relationships and make introverts valued confidants in times of need.

Creativity flourishes in the minds of many introverts, perhaps unexpectedly to some. Their preference for solitude creates the perfect environment for imagination and innovation to thrive. Free from the external noise, introverts can explore ideas deeply and uniquely, contributing to artistic, scientific, and logistical breakthroughs. History is peppered with introverted visionaries who have reshaped our world, using their solitary contemplation to revolutionize fields from science to art.

Introverts also excel in areas requiring persistence and resilience. Their cautious and thorough approach means they often remain committed to their goals despite setbacks. This persistence can lead to great accomplishments that require sustained effort and dedication. Introverts understand that success is often a long game, where endurance and steadfastness pay off in the end.

Another area where introverts shine is in analytical and strategic thinking. Their propensity for contemplation often leads them to consider multiple facets of a problem, weighing potential outcomes before reaching conclusions. This methodical thinking is an asset in planning and decision-making, ensuring that processes are both efficient and effective. Introverts may offer quiet but profound contributions to strategic discussions, often noticing details others might overlook.

Additionally, introverts exhibit a strong sense of independence. Comfortable with solitude, they often require less social validation and are more likely to forge their own paths. This independence allows introverts to pursue interests and projects aligned with their intrinsic motivations rather than the expectations of others. It's a quality that can lead to unique innovations and contributions to their fields.

Moreover, introverts tend to have a natural ability to notice nuances and subtleties in their environment. Their observant nature means they're adept at picking up on nonverbal cues and fine details, whether in personal interactions or broader professional contexts. This skill can be integral in negotiations, conflict resolutions, or any situation where understanding unspoken communication is crucial.

In concluding this overview of strengths, it's crucial to emphasize that introversion is not a trait to overcome; rather, it's a distinctive style of interacting with the world. For society to truly appreciate the fullness of humanity's potential, it must acknowledge and empower these quiet strengths. Only then can we hope to embrace the balanced and inclusive narrative that introverts deserve.

Debunking Myths Surrounding Introversion

Misunderstandings about introversion swirl around us like autumn leaves in the wind, often obscuring the profound beauty of quietude. Despite a growing awareness of introversion's value, myths persist, perpetuated by cultural norms that equate extroversion with success and charisma. It's time to sweep away these misconceptions and embrace the unique strengths that introverts offer the world.

One of the most pervasive myths is that introverts dislike people or are inherently anti-social. This myth can be both hurtful and limiting, trapping introverts in a narrative that doesn't reflect their reality. Introverts often crave deep, meaningful connections rather than surface-level interactions. While they might prefer a cozy night in with a small group of friends to a bustling party, this choice stems from a desire for authenticity, not avoidance.

Equally misleading is the idea that introverts lack practical skills in social situations. Underestimating introverts in networking or leadership scenarios misses the mark profoundly. Introverts possess a natural ability to listen, to truly hear, and understand the needs and expressions of those around them. In a world that often prioritizes talking over listening, this is a strength that can lead to profound and genuine connections.

The myth of introverts as shy or lacking confidence further mischaracterizes them. While some introverts might be shy, shyness isn't an introverted trait. It's a separate quality that some introverts and extroverts share. Importantly, introverts can be confident and assertive; their approach just might not involve dominating a conversation or a room. Their power often lies in thoughtful contemplation and quiet influence, characteristics that can reshape environments over time rather than single-handedly commanding attention.

Another assumption is that introverts don't make good leaders. Historically, leadership has been epitomized as a role suited for the brash, commanding presence of extroverts. However, research and real-world examples show the opposite can be true. Introverts often lead with empathy and thoughtfulness, fostering environments of collaboration, respect, and innovation. Leaders like Rosa Parks and Bill Gates epitomize how introspection and listening can translate into transformative leadership.

Introverts are also frequently assumed to be less creative than their extroverted counterparts, a notion easily dispelled by the works of countless contemplative geniuses. Creativity often blooms in solitude, where ideas have the space to be nurtured and reflect on their implications. Introverts excel in tapping into their inner worlds, drawing from a wellspring of reflection that can lead to groundbreaking innovations and deeply impactful art.

It's also crucial to address the myth that introverts can't enjoy or succeed in social gatherings and events. While their energy might deplete faster in a highly stimulating environment, it doesn't mean introverts can't revel in them or gain fulfillment. Strategies like finding quiet corners to recharge or engaging in smaller, more intimate conversations can allow introverts to not only endure but also enjoy social settings without compromising their energy needs.

The assumption that introversion is something to 'overcome' also needs reevaluation. Viewing introversion as a hurdle perpetuates unnecessary feelings of inadequacy and alienation. Instead, recognizing introversion as a spectrum that offers diverse strengths allows introverts to find and embrace roles that align with their natural inclinations. This shift in perspective can empower introverts to harness their unique capabilities rather than conforming to extroverted expectations.

The path towards debunking these myths isn't just about correction but also celebration. By embracing the full narrative of what it means to be introverted, we're reminded that introversion isn't a limitation but a vibrant, intrinsic part of human diversity. Each myth we debunk opens doors for introverts to contribute more freely and for society to benefit from the rich tapestry of introverted insights and abilities.

In challenging these misconceptions, we not only uplift introverts but enrich our collective understanding of human interaction. By recognizing, valuing, and nurturing the quiet power within, the myths obstructing the view gradually fade, revealing a landscape where introversion thrives not as an exception but as an integral part of a balanced world.

Chapter 3: The Evolution of Introverted Leaders

Embarking on the path of leadership has long been seen as the domain of the overtly confident and socially dominant, yet history tells a different story. Introverted leaders, though they may have often been overshadowed, have profoundly shaped the world with their unique strengths. Over time, they've demonstrated that quiet can indeed be powerful. Armed with deep listening skills, thoughtful planning, and an often underappreciated knack for empathy, these leaders have thrived by turning introspection into their greatest asset. Historical figures—those who preferred reflection over rhetoric—found ways to inspire through vision and authenticity rather than mere charisma. In today's rapidly changing world, the demand for such nuanced leadership has only intensified. Modern introverted leaders stand at the forefront of change, crafting strategies not through the roar of a crowd but the strength of keen insight and thoughtful dialogue. As society shifts its perspective, it increasingly recognizes the indispensable role these leaders play, thus celebrating the evolution of a leadership style that embraces introversion as an integral strength rather than a limitation.

Historical Figures Who Harnessed Introversion

The tapestry of history is woven with the threads of countless individuals whose quiet strength and reflective nature have propelled them to greatness. These are the introverted leaders who, despite the world's clamor for loudness, chose instead to lead with introspection, empathy, and resolve. Their stories offer not just inspiration but also valuable lessons on the power of embracing one's authentic self.

Take the revered American president, Abraham Lincoln. Known for his reflective demeanor and thoughtful decision-making, Lincoln utilized his introverted qualities to guide the nation through one of its darkest periods. His tendency to ponder deeply allowed him to weigh the complexities of preserving a fragmented nation. Through the filter of solitude, he crafted the Emancipation Proclamation, a testament to the profound influence of quiet leadership. Lincoln's legacy challenges the misconception that charisma and extroversion are prerequisites for leadership excellence.

Another exemplary figure is Mahatma Gandhi, whose life was a powerful testament to the strength of peaceful perseverance. Gandhi's introverted nature was evident in his preference for small gatherings and written communication over grand orations. His ability to listen deeply and reflect paved the way for a movement that changed the course of India's history. Gandhi's leadership style was not about dominating the conversation; instead, it was about empowering others through collective introspection and unwavering will, showing that steadfast resolve often stems from a quiet heart.

Albert Einstein, the physicist whose theories revolutionized our understanding of the universe, was famously introverted. He spent countless hours in solitude, allowing his mind to wander beyond conventional boundaries. These contemplative moments led to groundbreaking insights that extroverted interactions might have stifled. Einstein's story illustrates the notion that innovative ideas often blossom in the rich soil of quiet contemplation, a domain where introverts are uniquely poised to flourish.

The literary world provides further evidence of introversion's power. Jane Austen, author of iconic novels such as "Pride and Prejudice," used her profound observational skills to create characters and stories that remain relevant today. Austen's ability to immerse herself in the nuances of human relationships and societal dynamics was a direct extension of her introverted tendencies, which enabled her to write with unparalleled insight and empathy.

In the realm of art, one cannot overlook the influence of Vincent van Gogh. While his life was fraught with personal challenges, his introversion allowed him to channel his emotional depths into stunning works of art. Each brushstroke was a dialogue between his inner world and the canvas, revealing layers of complexity and emotional intensity. Van Gogh's legacy reminds us that great art often emerges from solitude and the profound explorations that only introverts dare to undertake.

Moreover, the world of music offers the story of J.S. Bach, whose intricate compositions are the result of hours spent in introspective solitude. Bach's life was not dominated by public performances or social engagements, but by a deep communion with his craft. The complexity and depth of his compositions reflect his introspective nature, illuminating the potential for introverts to touch the profoundest chords of the human soul through their work.

These historical figures, among many others, exemplify how introversion can be a formidable asset rather than a hindrance. They remind us that leadership and influence don't always manifest through bold oratory or public personas. Instead, the quiet reflection and intrinsic motivation that characterize introverted leaders can lead to significant and lasting impact.

Today's society often undervalues these traits, urging individuals to adopt more extroverted behaviors, but looking at history unfurls a different narrative. The enduring legacies of these introverted leaders challenge us to redefine leadership not by volume or visibility but by the virtue of thoughtful, intentional action.

As we draw inspiration from their journeys, it becomes clear that by embracing one's introverted nature, an individual can seamlessly blend personal authenticity with professional excellence. These leaders leveraged their natural dispositions to pioneer change and foster inspiration, proving that introversion is not an obstacle but a unique path to be explored and celebrated.

The stories of these historical figures serve not only as a profound acknowledgment of introverted power but also as a rallying cry for introverts today. To harness introversion is to accept its gifts: the ability to listen, to reflect, and to create with depth. History bears witness to the transformative potential of these attributes, urging us to embrace them in our quest to lead meaningful lives.

Modern Leaders and Their Introverted Traits

As we navigate the multifaceted landscape of modern leadership, it's increasingly evident that introverts have staked a formidable claim on the territory of influence and achievement. In a world often dominated by the clamor of extroversion, introverted leaders bring a refreshing, and often transformative, approach that merits celebration and emulation. Their rise isn't due to a shift in personality norms alone, but rather a testament to the strengths innate in introversion—traits that have been harnessed and adapted to today's challenges.

Consider some of the world's most innovative leaders—such as Bill Gates, Warren Buffet, and Barack Obama. These individuals embody the quiet power that introverts can unleash. Gates, for instance, is widely known for his contemplative nature, a trait that has enabled him to think strategically and anticipate future trends with a depth that often goes unnoticed by more gregarious counterparts. His ability to focus deeply and think methodically has been crucial to his success and the enduring impact of Microsoft. Through reflection and moments of solitude, introverted leaders find clarity and insight that propel their teams and organizations to thrive.

A hallmark of introverted leaders is their penchant for deep thought and intentional decision-making. Unlike their extroverted colleagues who often gain energy and ideas through interaction, introverted leaders typically prefer solitude to hone their strategic thinking. This is not to suggest that they shy away from collaboration; rather, they use their introspective processes to bring thoughtful, well-considered ideas to the table. This depth of processing fosters an environment where ideas are meticulously vetted, particularly advantageous in these times of rapid change and complexity.

The manner in which introverts approach leadership also reflects a profound resilience and empathy, often underappreciated in high-pressure environments. Warren Buffet's investment philosophy, for instance, exemplifies patience—a quintessentially introverted quality. His ability to remain calm and focused through turbulent market fluctuations has not only protected investments but strengthened the trust and dedication of those who follow his guidance. Here, we see introversion as an ally in cultivating resilience and insight, invaluable traits in uncertain times.

Introverted leaders also tend to exhibit a powerful, albeit understated, approach to communication. This approach emphasizes listening, an attribute that fosters co-operation and builds trust within teams. Take Barack Obama, whose presidency highlighted the power of listening and thoughtful dialogue. His reflective nature and keen ability to listen not only facilitated more inclusive policy developments but also encouraged a diverse array of voices to be heard and considered in the decision-making process. This empathetic leadership style is not only inspiring but essential in fostering inclusive and supportive environments that encourage collective success.

Moreover, introverted leaders often excel in creating environments where others are empowered to succeed. They possess a unique ability to elevate others, drawing out potential and creativity without overshadowing them. Marissa Mayer, former CEO of Yahoo!, exemplifies this trait. Known for her meticulous attention to detail, Mayer empowered her teams by creating space for innovation and fostering a culture that valued the unique contributions of each individual. This ability to inspire and cultivate a diverse range of talents speaks powerfully to the inclusivity of introverted leadership.

While it may seem that extroverts naturally fill leadership roles due to their visibility and dynamism, introverts often lead through influence rather than control. Their influence is borne out of respect and authenticity, generating a sense of stability and trust among their teams. This approach might not dominate headlines, but it builds enduring organizations that adapt and thrive over time.

These introverted traits aren't restrictive but expansive, encouraging leaders to draw strength from their natural inclinations rather than conforming to an extroverted mold. Through the celebration and harnessing of introversion, modern leaders can not only adapt to but flourish in today's fast-paced, complex world. The introverted leader's strength doesn't lie in seeking the spotlight, but in finding balance and depth within their leadership styles, which in turn creates resilient organizations poised for long-term success.

Ultimately, the current era of introverted leaders serves as a clarion call for authenticity and diversity in styles and approaches. Their introspective and resilient natures remind us that leadership doesn't have to be loud to be strong, nor flamboyant to be effective. By embracing the qualities that define them, introverts are redefining success, illustrating that the silent power they wield can lead to movements, innovations, and narratives that touch countless lives worldwide.

Chapter 4: Cultivating Self-Acceptance

In a world that often favors the outgoing and the outspoken, embracing one's introverted nature can feel daunting but is undeniably empowering. It's about recognizing that self-worth isn't measured by the volume of our voices but by the depth of our thoughts and the strength of our convictions. Introverts often face societal biases that mistakenly equate quietness with weakness, and overcoming these misconceptions begins with nurturing self-acceptance. By reorienting our inner compass, we learn to appreciate the unique strengths that come with introspection and thoughtful reflection. This journey of self-discovery isn't just about acceptance; it's about building an unshakeable confidence from within, recognizing that our quiet power holds immense potential. Each step towards self-acceptance is a step towards authenticity, allowing us to stand firm in who we are and to engage with the world on our terms. In doing so, we don't just change our perception of ourselves but also contribute to a broader narrative that values diversity in expression and thought.

Overcoming Societal Bias

Introverts often navigate a world that seems tailor-made for extroverts. In many cultures, the outgoing and gregarious are celebrated, while the quiet and reserved may feel overlooked. This societal bias can be challenging, but it's also an opportunity for change and growth. The journey toward self-acceptance for introverts begins by understanding and challenging these biases.

The very nature of introversion often leads to misunderstanding. Societal norms tend to prize extroverted behaviors like assertiveness and sociability. However, it's essential to recognize these are not inherent indicators of success or competency. Introverts have their unique strengths—introspection, deep focus, and thoughtfulness—that contribute equally to personal and professional success.

Research shows that introverts tend to process information differently than their extroverted peers, often reflecting before acting, which can lead to better decision-making. Yet, the subtle power of this introspection is often underestimated in cultures that associate action with progress. By recognizing and valuing these differences, we can begin to dismantle societal biases.

Language plays a significant role in shaping perception. Terms like "shy" or "reserved" are sometimes used pejoratively or as euphemisms for ineptness. Reframing the narrative around introversion is crucial for fostering an environment where all personality types are appreciated. Words like "thoughtful" or "intuitive" better capture the essence of what introverts bring to the table.

Overcoming societal bias involves both individual efforts and a collective shift in perspective. For introverts, building self-acceptance begins with recognizing their own value and contributions. Practice mindfulness and allow yourself to appreciate your unique qualities. This inner acknowledgment can serve as a buffer against external judgments.

From a societal standpoint, education and awareness are pivotal. Introversion is not a deficiency to be corrected, but a personality trait that can offer profound insights and contributions. By promoting awareness from early education through professional settings, we can nurture a balanced view that respects both introverted and extroverted personalities.

Challenging societal bias also involves highlighting stories of introverted individuals who have thrived in various fields. Their journeys and successes provide a counter-narrative to the prevailing stereotypes, demonstrating that introversion is not a barrier but a different path to achievement.

Finding allies in this journey is essential. Create or join communities that support introverted strengths. These networks offer validation and inspiration, fostering a sense of belonging and validation. Whether through support groups, online forums, or professional organizations, finding like-minded individuals helps reinforce self-acceptance and empowerment.

Introverts also have the opportunity to influence societal perspectives through advocacy. Whether by mentoring others, sharing personal stories, or participating in public discourse, actively engaging with the wider community can shift the narrative. Every conversation that raises awareness and understanding helps to normalize introversion as a valued aspect of human diversity.

In professional environments, advocating for more inclusive work cultures is critical. Introverts can thrive in settings that value deep work and quiet perseverance. Promoting flexible work arrangements, designed spaces for focused work, and valuing diverse communication styles can help create workplaces that recognize and harness the strengths of introverted employees.

Overcoming societal bias is as much about changing external perceptions as it is about cultivating inner acceptance. By embracing their introverted nature, individuals can align their internal values with their external actions. This congruence leads to authenticity, which is a powerful form of self-expression.

While societal bias won't disappear overnight, every small step towards acceptance counts. As more introverts embrace their strengths and contribute their unique perspectives, the social fabric will stretch to accommodate this diversity. In this enriched tapestry, introversion is not a detour but a vital part of human expression.

Ultimately, overcoming societal bias involves both educating extroverted peers and empowering introverts to celebrate their unique attributes. With every stride towards self-appreciation and challenging misconceptions, introverts contribute to a more inclusive society that values all voices, quiet or loud.

Building Confidence from Within

Finding confidence as an introvert often begins with a deep, internal journey. It's not about changing who you are to fit into a mold that society may idealize but about embracing your inherent qualities and recognizing the unique strengths you possess. For introverts, this means shifting the focus from external validation to internal solace and self-understanding, creating a foundation for authentic self-confidence.

Many introverts may feel challenged by the loudness of the world that seems to favor extroverted traits. Yet, true confidence emerges not from trying to be something you're not but from embracing your quiet power. Understanding your personal strengths, such as deep listening, empathy, and the ability to form meaningful one-on-one connections, can form the backbone of self-assurance that doesn't waver in the face of societal noise.

Introverts excel in self-reflection, an ability that forms a crucial part of building inner confidence. Reflecting on past experiences allows introverts to discern what environments empower them, which interactions drain them, and where their talents truly shine. This introspection isn't just a passive pastime; it's a strategic tool for understanding oneself deeply and recognizing one's worth beyond social expectations.

When you learn to value your own unique perspective, you're engaging in an act of self-acceptance that builds confidence. The key is to internalize the fact that your introversion isn't a hurdle or a setback. Rather, it's an integral part of who you are—an attribute that can lead to profound insights and thoughtful contributions in both personal and professional settings.

Setting personal goals based on your strengths can further enhance confidence from within. These goals should resonate with your inherent qualities, whether it's cultivating deeper connections, pursuing creative projects in solitude, or leading with a calm and steady presence. By aligning your ambitions with your authentic self, you're not only more likely to achieve them but do so in a way that reinforces your self-esteem.

Another vital component of internal confidence building is self-compassion. In a world that may often seem demanding, it's essential to treat yourself with kindness and understanding. Introverts might sometimes feel pressured to act against their nature to meet external expectations. Acknowledging these pressures without judgment and giving yourself grace as you navigate them can reinforce your inner strength.

Community can also play a critical role in building confidence for introverts. Finding a group of like-minded individuals who appreciate your quiet strengths can be immensely empowering. In such communities, you can share experiences, learn from others, and receive support without the expectation of conforming to extroverted norms. This camaraderie can remind you of your worth and solidify your sense of belonging.

Whether practicing mindfulness, engaging in journaling, or simply taking time for solitary reflection, cultivating mental spaces where you can recharge and center yourself is crucial. These practices serve as a reminder of the peace and clarity that can be found within, reinforcing your capacity to navigate life confidently, even when the external world feels overwhelming.

Introverts typically thrive in environments where they can work independently and express themselves in meaningful ways. Acknowledging and creating spaces that cater to these preferences can bolster self-confidence. Whether it's setting up a serene workspace at home or seeking out roles that allow for deep creative focus, tailoring your surroundings to your strengths can play a significant role in confidence-building.

Ultimately, building confidence from within as an introvert means honoring your intrinsic needs and values. It's about understanding that true self-acceptance is not dependent on others' perceptions or being the loudest voice in the room. Instead, it's about nurturing a deep-seated belief in your abilities and a resilient trust in your perspective.

As introverts begin to own their narrative, they not only change their internal dialogue but also influence how society views introversion. By exhibiting confidence in their natural demeanor, introverts contribute to shifting societal perspectives, illustrating that quiet strength can lead to profound success.

In conclusion, building confidence from within is a transformative journey that requires patience, practice, and a steadfast belief in oneself. For introverts, it's about celebrating the strengths that come with introspective and thoughtful nature while steadfastly working towards self-acceptance. Embrace your path, knowing it's an authentic reflection of who you are—a journey not merely towards confidence but towards an empowered existence in every facet of life.

Chapter 5: Career Success for Introverts

In the bustling world of careers, where the spotlight often favors extroverted charisma, introverts can find unexpected paths to success by leveraging their innate strengths. Rather than blending in with a culture that glorifies gregariousness, introverts thrive by choosing roles that align with their reflective nature, bringing depth and insight into their work environments. This chapter peels back the bias-ridden fabric of office culture, showing how introverts can navigate politics not with loud voices but through quiet strength and strategic action. Harnessing patience, focus, and empathy allows introverts to excel while staying true to themselves. The journey to career fulfillment involves understanding one's preferences and utilizing them to sculpt a satisfying profession—one that not only respects but celebrates the introverted nature. Success doesn't demand being the loudest in the room; it requires authenticity, a keen understanding, and the confidence to walk a unique path. Introverts possess these qualities and more, setting the stage for a fulfilling career woven with quiet triumph.

Choosing Careers Aligned with Introversion

Choosing a career that resonates with one's inner nature is not only liberating but also crucial for long-term success and satisfaction. For introverts, this often means finding vocations that embrace their natural strengths rather than forcing them to adopt extroverted personas that don't feel authentic. In a world that often seems built for the gregarious, introverts possess unique attributes—deep focus, thoughtful decision-making, and an innate ability to listen—that can be impeccably matched to certain career paths.

Understanding your own preferences is the foundational step in seeking a career aligned with introversion. This involves an honest assessment of what environments energize or drain you, where your passions lie, and how you respond to different types of interactions and settings. While societal norms may urge you to pursue traditionally 'successful' roles in high-stakes, team-driven environments, it's crucial to discern what truly aligns with your personal and professional goals.

Many introverts thrive in roles that allow them to work independently or in small groups, where profound thinking and creativity are valued over constant networking and socializing. Fields like writing, research, design, accounting, and technology offer environments that cater to these preferences. In these roles, introverts can often delve deeply into projects, strategize without disruption, and innovate with clarity.

Take, for example, the world of technology and software development. This industry often celebrates the solitary deep work that allows introverts to shine. Programmers and developers can find significant satisfaction in coding for hours without the need for continuous social engagement. Such roles capitalize on meticulous problem-solving skills and the ability to foresee long-term outcomes—qualities that are naturally embedded in many introverts.

Art and design are other avenues where introverts frequently excel. These fields appreciate the ability to work independently and the need for solitude in the creative process. Whether through visual arts, music composition, or graphic design, introverts can express their thoughts and emotions in ways that resonate profoundly, both with themselves and with audiences.

Introverts also often find fulfillment in roles that center around analysis and observation. Positions in scientific research, data analysis, and librarianship allow for a deep dive into subjects without the demand for constant collaboration. Here, introverts can focus on detail-oriented tasks that harness their ability to concentrate and analyze complex information critically.

While many introverts gravitate towards roles traditionally considered as solitary, it's important to note that they can thrive in leadership positions as well. The key is finding environments that appreciate the strengths introverts bring to the table—such as empathy, reflective thinking, and the ability to listen and understand deeply before acting.

Management roles that emphasize one-on-one communication and foster a supportive atmosphere can be ideal for introverted leaders. Here, they can leverage their strengths to build strong relationships with team members and encourage an inclusive, respectful work culture. By focusing on quiet strength, introverts in these roles can influence profound change and inspire loyalty among those they lead.

Ultimately, the choice lies in creating a career path that resonates with one's authentic self. This often requires creativity in how career goals are pursued. Being an introvert doesn't mean you're limited to a particular set of jobs. Instead, it's about tailoring one's strengths to fit a myriad of potential roles.

Exploring unconventional career paths can also unlock unexpected opportunities. For instance, roles in nature and outdoors, like park rangers or conservation scientists, allow introverts to work autonomously while being deeply connected to nature. These positions often require self-motivation and the ability to work independently—qualities that many introverts bring naturally.

Recognizing and pursuing passions are also significant aspects of choosing an introvert-aligned career. Whether it's harnessing a hobby into a freelance career or turning a love for literature into a profession in publishing, following one's interests can often lead to fulfilling, long-term career satisfaction.

Introverts might also consider entrepreneurship as a viable path. It may seem daunting, but many introverts excel at it because it allows complete control over social interactions and work environments. The ability to create a business that reflects personal values and working styles means that introverts can build enterprises where their traits are not just accepted but celebrated.

It's important for introverts to remember that career success doesn't require being someone they're not. By aligning career choices with their true selves, introverts not only enhance personal happiness but also bring invaluable contributions to diverse fields. Finding this alignment often means tuning out the buzz of societal expectations and listening carefully to one's internal compass.

In conclusion, choosing a career aligned with introversion involves more than just picking a job. It's about understanding and embracing strengths, acknowledging personal preferences, and involving oneself in work that feels meaningful and rewarding. The path may not always be straightforward, but it is undeniably transformative, leading to a fulfilling professional life that empowers introverts to thrive authentically.

Navigating Office Politics with Quiet Strength

Introverts often find themselves navigating the intricate web of office politics with a sense of trepidation. It's a world seemingly crafted for extroverts, where being loud and seen is sometimes mistaken for leadership. But within this bustling environment, introverts have a unique edge—the capacity to observe, reflect, and choose actions thoughtfully. Harnessing these strengths can transform the daunting task of office politics into an opportunity for personal and professional growth.

At its core, office politics are about relationships and influence. Contrary to the perception that only the outspoken can sway decisions, introverts are adept at understanding team dynamics. Their attentive nature allows them to perceive the undercurrents of workplace interactions that can easily be missed by those who are always in the limelight. Instead of positioning oneself as the loudest person in the room, introverts can opt to build alliances based on genuine understanding and trust. Empathy becomes a superpower, enabling introverts to form connections that are both deep and lasting.

For introverts, recognizing the value of their listening skills is crucial. While others may rush to voice their opinions, introverts can lead by listening first and speaking second. By doing so, they capture the essence of discussions, identify what truly matters to their colleagues, and contribute thoughts that are both timely and relevant. It's a quiet form of leadership that compels others to listen when the introvert eventually speaks, often leading to more profound and meaningful exchanges.

Moreover, introverts excel at strategic thinking—a remarkable asset when navigating office politics. In meetings or decision-making scenarios, their approach is to weigh options carefully, consider different perspectives, and propose solutions that harmonize competing interests. Through this considered approach, introverts can guide discussions towards resolutions that benefit the collective, reinforcing their position as pivotal players within their organizations.

There's an understated charisma in wielding what can be termed as "quiet strength." Instead of engaging in power plays, introverts often choose to contribute through collaborative leadership, focusing on fostering a sense of teamwork and shared purpose. By supporting peers and encouraging a culture of open dialogue, introverts create a work environment where each team member feels valued, ultimately leading to a more cohesive unit.

Another powerful tactic for introverts is leveraging their natural inclination for thoughtfulness to build influence gradually. In team settings, they can shine by acknowledging colleagues' contributions and making them feel heard. This subtle nod of recognition does not only strengthen interpersonal ties but also paves the way for introverts to be seen as fair, insightful, and wise leaders in workplace settings.

In encounters where traditional politicking feels unavoidable, introverts can rely on their introspective nature to devise strategies. Knowing when to engage and when to retreat is key. For instance, it might be beneficial to step back from heated discussions and revisit them with calm and reason later. This ability to pause and regroup helps prevent hasty decisions and ensures that actions taken are aligned with both personal integrity and company values.

Building a network quietly but effectively is another strength that introverts can lean into. Unlike extroverts who may prefer the energy of large social gatherings, introverts can create circles of influence through targeted and meaningful interactions. Whether it's a one-on-one coffee conversation or a well-crafted email, these personalized connections can resonate deeply and lead to professional acquaintances who are genuinely invested in mutual success.

Also, introverts often find strength in preparation. Prior to meetings or presentations, conducting thorough research and planning responses can turn potential vulnerabilities into advantages. Here, the quality of contributions outweighs the quantity, and being well-prepared reflects an impressive depth of knowledge and commitment.

Perhaps most importantly, introverts should honor their unique rhythms and find balance in work-life dynamics. Ensuring spaces for respite and reflection allows for recharging, making introverts more resilient when navigating the complexities of the office environment. It's essential for maintaining the stamina to approach office politics with grace and poise.

Celebrating introversion as a strength rather than a hurdle shifts the narrative of what office politics means. It underscores the potential for quiet leadership, driven not by self-promotion but by results and respectful influence. In doing so, introverts not only find their place within organizational hierarchies but redefine what success looks like in the modern workplace.

In embracing the power of their quiet strength, introverts inspire a broader move towards more inclusive professional environments, where diverse approaches to leadership and success are not just acknowledged but celebrated. This subtle yet profound shift can lead to more equitable workplaces that thrive on varied voices contributing to a shared purpose. By fostering an atmosphere where introverted qualities are recognized, introverts don't just navigate office politics—they transform it.

Chapter 6: Effective Communication for Introverts

In the vibrant cacophony of today's world, introverts often find the art of communication to be a complex dance, where their natural inclinations may seem overshadowed by louder voices. Yet, it's in these very nuances of introspection and thoughtful engagement that introverts possess a unique edge. Effective communication for introverts is not about transforming into someone they're not, but instead harnessing their strengths in deep listening, empathy, and the ability to foster genuine connections. By embracing their authentic selves, introverts can learn to master conversations with confidence, striking a balance between speaking up and thoughtful listening. Strategies such as preparation for public speaking or using one-on-one interactions to their advantage can further empower introverts to express their ideas compellingly. Through this, the quiet strength of introverted individuals has the potential to ignite discussions, build meaningful relationships, and influence change in personal and professional spheres.

Mastering Conversations with Confidence

Imagine walking into a room where conversations flow effortlessly around you, like a river of words you wish you could just swim into. For many introverts, this setting can cause anxiety, but there's something comforting to know: it's possible to master conversations with confidence. Conversation is not just about speaking; it's about connecting, understanding, and sharing. Introverts have unique strengths that can make them not only participants in conversations but masters of them.

One key to mastering conversations is preparation. While it might not sound spontaneous, being prepared can alleviate much of an introvert's anxiety about conversations. When you know what interests you, what topics you're passionate about, or even current events that spark your curiosity, you walk into interactions with a toolkit of ideas ready to be shared. Planning doesn't mean memorizing lines—it's about equipping yourself with knowledge and comfort in topics that resonate with you. With this foundation, you can steer conversations toward areas where you feel knowledgeable and comfortable.

Listening, often seen as a passive skill, is actually a power tool in conversations for introverts. Contrary to the myth that you must dominate a conversation to control it, listening allows you to guide it from a position of strength and empathy. When you listen actively, you hear not just words but emotions and intentions. This creates a deeper understanding and a connection that many extroverts might miss as they race through thoughts and dialogues. By honing your listening skills, you not only show people you value their words but also gather insights that inform your responses, making them more impactful and considered.

Moreover, asking open-ended questions can significantly enhance your conversational experience. These questions invite others to share more, keeping the conversation flowing without requiring extroverted energy from you. Questions that start with "how" or "why" encourage expansive answers and can subtly shift the focus away from you, allowing for more listening and learning from the person you're engaging with. This approach not only helps build a conversation naturally but also elevates your standing as an engaged and thoughtful interlocutor.

Confidence in conversations also stems from the ability to embrace pauses. Silence often carries a negative connotation, signaling awkwardness or a lack of things to say. However, introverts can redefine this notion. Pauses can give you the space to think, reflect, and then respond with clarity and purpose. It turns conversations into a dance rather than a sprint, where every step—every word—is deliberate. Recognizing that you don't have to fill every silence with chatter gives you power over the pace and depth of your interactions.

Understanding your energy levels is another crucial factor in conversational confidence for introverts. Since social interactions can be draining, it's important to know when to engage and when to retreat to recharge. Planning your interactions around times when you feel your best can make a significant difference. Don't hesitate to politely bow out when you need a break. People respect boundaries, and learning to communicate your needs clearly—and without guilt—is part of building your conversational prowess.

Another effective technique is the art of storytelling. Introverts are often natural storytellers due to their reflective nature. When you tell stories, you share pieces of yourself in a narrative that captivates and connects with others. Stories humanize data, facts, and ideas, carrying an emotional weight that resonates. They don't have to be epic or involve grand adventures; they can be simple anecdotes that convey personal truths and lessons. Mastering this art allows you to communicate in a way that leaves lasting impressions.

It's essential to remember that it's okay to offer your perspective in parts or fragments, emphasizing your point of view gradually. Introverts often benefit from reflecting before sharing their thoughts. This measured sharing not only gives you room to craft thoughtful responses but signals to others your contemplative strength, inviting them into a richer dialogue.

Building conversational confidence also involves overcoming the fear of being judged, which often stems from internalized societal biases that favor extroversion. It's crucial to remind yourself that your perspective is valuable and deserving of space. You bring depth and insight to conversations that might not be immediately visible but are profoundly impactful when shared. By affirming your worth in every interaction, over time, confidence becomes second nature.

Inclusion in conversations is another area where introverts can shine. Being the one to draw others in who might also feel overlooked fosters a more inclusive dialogue. It shows leadership and humility, endearing you to those who benefit from your openness. This not only builds your network but enriches conversations through diverse perspectives.

Finally, embracing technology can bolster your conversational confidence. Digital communication offers introverts time to reflect and formulate their thoughts without the pressure of immediate response. Platforms like forums or social media can help introverts practice interactions, explore ideas, and develop their voice in a space that accommodates their rhythm. This kind of practice translates back into face-to-face interactions, enhancing overall communication skills.

In mastering conversations with confidence, you aren't changing who you are; you're amplifying the strengths that make you, as an introvert, uniquely powerful in dialogue. Each step you take toward comfortable and meaningful interaction strengthens the broader narrative that introspective voices are vital and impactful in every sphere of life. Through preparation, active listening, thoughtful questioning, and embracing your narrative style, you craft conversations that are not only confident but profoundly enriching.

Strategies for Public Speaking

For many introverts, the thought of public speaking can evoke a mix of dread and discomfort. However, public speaking doesn't have to be a daunting endeavor. With the right strategies, introverts can excel on stage, transforming what might feel like a personal challenge into an opportunity for growth and influence. It all begins with understanding the unique strengths that introverts bring to the table.

Introverts often possess a deep well of knowledge on subjects they are passionate about, allowing them to offer insightful perspectives that engage audiences. Before stepping onto a stage, consider consuming information and immersing yourself in the topic you're about to present. The more connected you are with the material, the more you're likely to convey confidence and authority—a key factor in capturing an audience's attention.

Preparation is an introvert's best friend. Unlike extroverts, who may thrive in spontaneous situations, introverts often benefit from planning and rehearsing. Begin by outlining the key points you wish to communicate, organizing them into a coherent and compelling narrative. Practice your speech out loud, preferably in front of a mirror or a trusted friend who can provide constructive feedback. Repetition builds familiarity, helping to reduce anxiety and enhance delivery.

Visual aids, such as slides or props, can serve as an effective buffer between the speaker and the audience, providing a focal point that alleviates the pressure of constant eye contact. Use visuals to reinforce your message and maintain the audience's engagement. By channeling your focus towards the visuals, you allow your innate capacity for introspection and analysis to shine through, distilling complex ideas into digestible content.

The physical space in which you present also plays a crucial role. Arriving early at the venue allows you to acclimate to the environment and make necessary adjustments. Familiarize yourself with the stage or podium, practice projection in the given space, and determine the most comfortable position for delivering your speech. Sometimes, a simple stroll across the stage can calm nerves and create a dynamic interaction with the audience.

Breathing techniques can work miracles in mitigating anxiety. Introverts tend to default to shallow breathing under stress, which can exacerbate nervousness. Engage in deep, diaphragmatic breathing before and during your speech to maintain composure. By slowing your breath, you activate the body's relaxation response, which helps in modulating your heart rate and soothing pre-performance jitters.

It's important to remember that the audience is usually on your side. They are there to listen, learn, and engage with you and your topic. Embrace this understanding to shift the focus away from your nerves and towards the value you offer. The more you internalize that the audience is receptive rather than judgmental, the more natural your delivery will become, enhancing the overall communication experience.

Storytelling is a powerful tool at your disposal. Introverts excel at contemplation, often producing richly detailed inner narratives. Tap into these stories, sharing personal anecdotes or real-life examples to forge an emotional connection with your listeners. Stories not only anchor your message in tangible reality but also humanize the speaker, making the presentation memorable and impactful.

After speaking, involve the audience by opening the floor for questions or inviting feedback. This interaction can transform a monologue into a dialogue, making the experience more collaborative and less intimidating for introverts. View this as an extension of your presentation—an opportunity to delve deeper into topics of interest, correcting misunderstandings, and further building on your rapport with the audience.

Embrace nervousness rather than resisting it entirely. A modicum of anxiety sharpens focus and energizes your delivery if channeled effectively. Identify small rituals that ground you, whether it's wearing a favorite accessory, holding a stress ball, or simply taking a moment for silent reflection. These routines serve as psychological anchors, providing comfort and routine amidst the unpredictability of public speaking.

Finally, align your mindset with growth rather than perfection. Shifting your mental framework from fearing mistakes to seeing them as learning opportunities can transform your public speaking experience. Embrace the idea that every presentation is a stepping-stone towards mastery, fostering resilience and adaptability in your communication skills.

In conclusion, public speaking offers introverts the chance to exercise their quiet power in a domain traditionally perceived as extroverted. It is through meticulous preparation, deep understanding, and the strategic use of introverted strengths that introverts can redefine what it means to be an effective and inspiring speaker. Every voice must be heard, and introverts possess a wealth of wisdom that the world urgently needs.

Chapter 7: Building Meaningful Relationships

Building meaningful relationships as an introvert involves embracing the power of depth over breadth. While extroverts might thrive in large social circles, introverts often find true satisfaction in fostering a few genuine, deep connections. These relationships are nurtured through authentic communication and the willingness to be vulnerable, which can lead to profound bonds that are both fulfilling and empowering. By setting respectful boundaries, introverts protect their energy while creating space for connections that resonate on a deeper level. Empathy and active listening are key, allowing introverts to connect with others in a way that's both sincere and impactful. As introverts learn to balance solitude with the enriching experiences found in meaningful relationships, they discover that these bonds not only bring joy but also serve as a crucial support network in personal and professional settings. This journey offers a unique opportunity for introverts to redefine how they connect—proving that strength, love, and understanding can blossom in the quietest of spaces.

Forming Deep Connections

Introverts often find themselves pondering the nature of human connections more deeply than their extroverted counterparts. This isn't just about mingling or exchanging pleasantries; it's about truly understanding, feeling, and connecting on a profound level. Deep connections are the lifeblood of meaningful relationships and, for introverts, quality reigns over quantity. How, then, do introverts form these connections without compromising their essence?

To start, embracing authenticity is key. Introverts excel in environments where genuine expression is encouraged and valued. They avoid superficial interactions, choosing instead to share themselves only where they feel safe and understood. This means beginning relationships with an honesty that might seem daunting but is ultimately rewarding. When introverts engage with authenticity, they invite others to do the same, setting the stage for deeper bonds.

Active listening is another cornerstone of forming deep connections. Introverts have the innate ability to listen intently and process information with great depth. Where others might feel compelled to speak, introverts absorb. This skill ensures that when introverts do engage in conversation, they offer insights and perspectives rich in understanding. By listening, they not only gather information but also build a foundation of trust and empathy, which are crucial for deep connections.

- Choose environments that foster genuine interaction.
- Engage in conversations with intentionality and presence.
- Utilize their strength in empathy to relate to others on a personal level.

Investing in a few significant relationships rather than numerous superficial ones is another strategy introverts often employ. The energy it takes to maintain relationships can be overwhelming for introverts, so they choose to focus on a select few. These relationships are cultivated slowly over time, with mutual respect and understanding at their core.

Quality interactions, rather than frequent but shallow encounters, are what introverts seek. They thrive on the substance of shared ideas, values, and emotions.

The capacity for introspection gives introverts an edge in forming lasting bonds. They often reflect on their own feelings and behaviors, striving to understand not only themselves but their place in their relationships. This perspective allows introverts to be adaptive; they can consider how their actions and words affect those they care about, leading to more harmonious interactions. Through introspection, introverts can also identify areas of personal growth that might enhance their relationships further.

Despite their preference for solitude, introverts value community deeply. They may prefer smaller gatherings or one-on-one interactions, but this doesn't diminish their appreciation for the connections they form. In fact, introverts often nurture relationships that are as fulfilling as they are enduring. They are the friends who remember the important details, the colleagues who offer support during challenging times, and the partners who truly know their loved ones. This strong sense of community emerges from a lifetime of thoughtful investment in others.

Setting boundaries is a vital component of maintaining deep connections for introverts. Knowing when to retreat and recharge ensures that introverts can return to their relationships refreshed and engaged. Boundaries protect the depth of the connections by preventing overwhelm and burnout. Clear communication about personal needs isn't just a self-preservation tactic; it's an expression of respect for the relationship's health. Introverts can still be deeply connected without being constantly available, making boundaries a necessary groundwork for fostering relationships that last.

In forming deep connections, introverts must navigate not only their internal world but also the external perceptions and expectations of society. This journey requires courage and resilience. As introverts dare to be themselves, they pave the way for others to understand the richness they bring to their relationships. The quiet, introspective approach of introverts often reveals the most profound insights, fostering connections that are as meaningful as they are rare.

So, how does one navigate the intricacies of forming deep connections in a world that often seems louder than one's thoughts? It involves balancing the need for solitude with the desire for connection, embracing one's unique strengths in listening and empathy, and courageously seeking out authentic interactions. In doing so, introverts can build meaningful relationships that not only enrich their own lives but also inspire those around them to seek depth over breadth.

The journey to forming deep connections is a testament to the power and significance of introversion itself. It's a reminder that being introverted doesn't equate to being alone; rather, it's about finding those rare and precious connections that resonate at the deepest levels of our souls. In these relationships, introverts find not only companionship but a profound sense of belonging as well.

Setting Boundaries with Respect

Building meaningful relationships isn't just about understanding others; it's also about understanding yourself. For introverts, laying down boundaries can be both a protective measure and a path to deeper connections. In a world that often equates sociability with success, introverts might find the notion of boundaries as an empowering way to protect their energy without withdrawing completely. Establishing them with respect ensures that these boundaries are appreciated rather than resented, strengthening relationships rather than straining them.

Respectful boundaries start with self-awareness. Introverts need time to recharge, much like a battery needs to plug in to continue functioning. Recognizing what activities drain or refresh you can guide how you prioritize your time. Once you have this awareness, communicating these needs with clarity and kindness becomes essential. It's not about pushing people away but about inviting them to understand you better. For instance, you might inform a friend that while you cherish your time together, you also value your alone time for decompression and reflection.

Finding the right language to express your boundaries can make all the difference. It's easy to fall into the trap of feeling guilty or selfish, but boundaries tell a story about your needs, not your shortcomings. Phrases like "I need some time to myself after a busy day" or "I'm looking forward to spending time with you, but I need to recharge first" frame boundaries as a personal necessity rather than a rejection. Using "I" statements emphasizes that these needs are about you, reducing the chances of others feeling blamed or excluded.

Successful boundaries aren't one-time declarations; they're conversations that evolve with time and context. Life situations change, as do relationships. An introvert might need more downtime during a stressful period or may find they're comfortable with more social interactions when they've had ample rest. Keeping lines of communication open ensures that boundaries are fluid, not rigid walls. Regularly checking in with yourself and your loved ones about these boundaries helps maintain balance and mutual respect.

Integrating boundaries into professional relationships is equally crucial. Introverts may find that work environments can be particularly draining due to their inherent demand for collaboration and constant communication. Setting boundaries in a workplace starts with understanding your peak productivity times and preferred modes of interaction. It might involve scheduling uninterrupted work time or requesting to join meetings via calls instead of in a bustling conference room.

Communicating these preferences can be daunting in professional settings, but doing so confidently and respectfully can often be met with understanding. Rather than framing requests with an apologetic tone, using positive language to present your needs can foster a more collaborative atmosphere. Saying "I do my best work with some quiet focus time. Could we schedule meetings around this?" not only asserts your boundary but also shows your commitment to your work and responsibilities.

Ultimately, boundaries serve to protect the inner life of an introvert and enhance their external interactions. They create a space where introverts can maintain their serenity while participating meaningfully in their relationships. This delicate dance requires patience, honesty, and sometimes the courage to say no. It's about placing value on that inner world without diminishing one's capacity to engage authentically with others.

The beauty of respectful boundaries is that they invite others to reciprocate. It encourages an environment where everyone feels permitted to express their needs, creating a culture of mutual understanding and support. When others see you honor your own needs, they might feel more comfortable expressing their own, paving the way for more honest and fulfilling interactions.

Introverts possess a deep well of thought and empathy, which can be amplified in relationships when boundaries are respected rather than broken. When your boundaries are embraced, it not only reaffirms your self-worth but also enhances the depth of your connections with others. This respect for individual needs builds trust and fosters relationships that thrive on authenticity.

It's important to model and practice these principles with understanding and patience. Not everyone will immediately grasp the importance or nuances of your boundaries, but with time and gentle persistence, it becomes easier for others to see them as a pathway to a more harmonious relationship. With each interaction, you're contributing to a wider shift in how introversion and personal space are perceived.

As you continue to navigate personal and professional landscapes, remember that boundaries aren't barriers—they're bridges that can lead to richer, more meaningful connections. They serve as reminders that every relationship involves two dynamic individuals, each with their own rhythms and needs. Embrace this duality, and you'll find that boundaries set with respect can lead to newfound strengths in both yourself and your relationships.

Chapter 8: The Introvert's Approach to Leadership

Introverted leaders bring an authenticity to leadership that can often transform teams and organizations in profound ways. Their approach is characterized by deep listening, thoughtfulness, and a genuine appreciation for diverse perspectives. By leveraging their natural strengths, such as empathy and adaptability, introverted leaders create environments where team members feel valued and heard. Unlike the often loud and commanding stereotypical leadership styles, introverts lead with quiet confidence, making decisions based on careful reflection and fostering collaborative atmospheres. This method not only encourages innovation but also strengthens team dynamics by allowing space for individual contributions to shine. Introverted leaders show us that leadership isn't about fitting into a predefined mold but about embracing and utilizing one's unique qualities to inspire and guide others towards common goals.

Leading Teams with Authenticity

Introverts often feel a strong resonance with authenticity, using it as a compass to navigate their leadership style. Unlike more extroverted approaches that might rely heavily on outward expressions and charisma, introverted leaders draw strength from their inner world, allowing them to lead with integrity and purpose. It's this authenticity that can forge genuine connections with team members, creating an atmosphere of trust and mutual respect.

Leading with authenticity means embracing one's true self and being transparent about strengths and weaknesses. Introverted leaders can excel here as their inward-focused nature often results in a high level of self-awareness. They pay attention to their values, are mindful of their actions, and listen deeply, qualities that are key in developing a coherent and genuine leadership style. Sharing personal stories or experiences can be a powerful way for leaders to communicate their journey. This openness can humanize the leader, making them more relatable and trustworthy.

One might ask, how does an introverted leader effectively manage a team without the loud presence that's often associated with leadership success? The answer lies in leading from behind the scenes. Introverts have a knack for observing and listening, picking up nuances that might be missed by others. This careful attention allows them to understand team dynamics fully and anticipate issues before they arise. By addressing these quietly and efficiently, introverted leaders can make significant impacts without needing to dominate conversations or meetings.

Authenticity in leadership isn't just about being true to oneself; it's also about empowering others to do the same. Introverted leaders tend to be less interested in personal accolades and more focused on the collective success of their teams. They often foster environments where team members feel encouraged to share ideas and take ownership of their contributions. This empowerment can lead to increased morale, innovation, and collaboration, hallmarks of a thriving team.

Moreover, the introverted approach to authenticity involves a deep-seated commitment to listening. When introverted leaders listen, it's not just about absorbing information. It's about understanding and valuing the perspectives of their team members. This practice builds a culture of inclusion and recognition, where every voice feels heard and respected. By giving others the space to express their thoughts and ideas, introverted leaders can facilitate a rich diversity of perspectives, leading to better problem-solving and more innovative outcomes.

Another key element of leading authentically is consistency. Team members who see their leader consistently acting in alignment with their stated values and beliefs gain confidence in leadership. For introverts, this consistency is a natural extension of their preference for consistency and depth over breadth. Their leadership is often marked by a steady and calm presence, providing stability in times of change or uncertainty. This can be immensely reassuring for team members, allowing them to focus on their work without unnecessary distractions or anxieties.

But leading with authenticity isn't without its challenges, especially in environments that might favor extroverted leadership styles. Introverted leaders may feel pressured to adapt or change their approach to fit a more traditional mold. However, it's crucial for introverted leaders to resist the urge to conform at the expense of their authentic self. Instead, they can lean into their introverted strengths and demonstrate how these qualities bring value to their leadership approach.

One strategy is to establish clear communication channels and expectations from the outset. This ensures that team members understand the introverted leader's approach and feel comfortable interacting with them. Open and honest communication is a cornerstone of authentic leadership, as it reinforces trust and transparency within the team. Introverted leaders can use written communication, such as thoughtful emails or notes, to effectively convey their vision and feedback, complementing more traditional spoken meetings.

Furthermore, building a leadership style focused on personal growth is another aspect of authenticity in introverted leadership. Introverted leaders often encourage ongoing learning and improvement, both for themselves and their teams. They model a growth mindset that values curiosity and encourages team members to explore their interests and develop new skills. This focus on development not only enhances team capabilities but also boosts team morale and engagement.

Introverted leaders can also benefit from surrounding themselves with complementary personalities. Recognizing the strengths and weaknesses of both themselves and their team members allows introverted leaders to form a balanced and effective team. For example, pairing with extroverted colleagues might help enhance outreach and engagement, while introverts can excel in strategic planning and reflection. This balance ensures a holistic approach to leadership, leveraging the best of both worlds.

Ultimately, leading teams with authenticity isn't about an introverted leader trying to mimic extroverted traits, but rather about embracing their inherent characteristics. This genuine approach not only empowers introverted leaders but also challenges the conventional notions of leadership, demonstrating that diverse styles can achieve extraordinary results. By staying true to themselves, introverted leaders can cultivate workplaces that are inclusive, innovative, and resilient, paving the way for sustainable success.

Leveraging Introverted Qualities in Management

Imagine a workplace where calm contemplation and deep listening are celebrated as vital leadership skills. It's a space where the quiet strength of introverts isn't just acknowledged but is harnessed to drive teams forward. For many, the concept of an introverted manager might seem like an oxymoron, given the long-held societal notion that leaders need to be outspoken and boisterous. Yet, in reality, introverts bring to the table a unique set of qualities that can transform the way teams operate and how success is achieved.

Introverted managers are often deeply focused and thoughtful individuals who make decisions after thorough consideration. Their ability to process information internally means that they can analyze complex problems and develop innovative solutions. This quality, known as reflective thinking, can be a significant asset in management, especially in today's fast-paced and information-heavy environments. Decision-making that's rooted in deep analysis rather than impulse can lead to more sustainable and effective outcomes.

Empathy, another hallmark of introverted leaders, allows them to connect with their teams on a more personal level. Introverts tend to be good listeners, providing a safe space for team members to voice concerns and share ideas. In management roles, this translates to building trust and fostering a cooperative and inclusive work atmosphere. When employees feel heard, their engagement and productivity levels naturally increase, which is a testament to the power of empathy in leadership.

Moreover, introverts often excel in one-on-one interactions, which can be pivotal in personnel management. These focused encounters give introverted leaders a chance to mentor, offer support, and provide feedback in a setting that suits their natural communication style. This approach doesn't just benefit the individual; it slowly but surely strengthens the fabric of the entire team. As employees grow and develop under such guidance, the organization's culture becomes one of mutual respect and growth.

The ability to manage through observant leadership is another understated yet potent introvert quality. Introverted leaders often excel at picking up on subtleties within team dynamics, recognizing shifts in morale, or identifying potential conflicts before they escalate. Their observational skills allow them to address issues discreetly and effectively, maintaining a harmonious work environment where potential disruptions are swiftly and silently handled. This creates a stable foundation where teams can thrive without unnecessary friction.

Crucially, introverted managers are also known for creating spaces that empower deep work. They recognize and respect the need for solitude and uninterrupted time, understanding that creative and impactful work often requires these conditions. By fostering an environment where focus is valued over constant interaction or multitasking, they enable their teams to achieve a level of productivity that might otherwise be difficult to reach.

One challenge that introverted managers might face is the need to navigate the extroverted norms prevalent in many corporate cultures. Yet, this is where the introvert's resilience shines. Rather than conforming to these norms, introverted leaders can redefine what it means to lead by example. They can demonstrate that adaptability and versatility in management styles, instead of fitting a single mold, can lead to a more balanced and effective leadership model.

Transparent communication, albeit in a calm and composed manner, is often a profound strength of introverted managers. They're not inclined to speak for the sake of speaking but choose their words wisely and with purpose. Such leaders are often clear and straightforward in their communication, which ensures that their message is understood without the noise of unnecessary rhetoric. It's a skill that facilitates clarity and minimizes misunderstandings, fostering a productive and efficient team dynamic.

In conclusion, leveraging introverted qualities in management isn't about changing who you are to fit a predefined role. It's about embracing those intrinsic traits that can lead to authentic and impactful leadership. The introverted approach acknowledges the strengths of deep thought, empathy, observation, and focused communication as elements that don't just succeed within a leadership framework—they reshape it. By valuing what introverts naturally bring to the table, organizations not only widen the leadership pool but also pave the way for a more inclusive, reflective, and effective working world. Through this lens, introverted managers are not only recognized but become indispensable architects of modern leadership. The quiet power of introversion, when harnessed effectively, has the potential to redefine what it means to lead.

Chapter 9: Enhancing Productivity and Creativity

In the heart of introspection lies a powerful catalyst for both productivity and creativity, two elements often underestimated in their potential symbiosis. Introverts, with their innate ability to relish solitude, possess a unique advantage: the power to transform quiet reflection into groundbreaking ideas and meticulously crafted projects. By creating personal workspaces that resonate with tranquility and inspiration, introverts can cultivate an environment where their thoughts flow freely, unencumbered by the usual distractions. In these sanctuaries, solitude thrives not as isolation but as fertile ground for innovation, allowing the mind to wander unfettered and discover connections often missed in the clamor of extroverted spaces. This harmony between productive output and creative exploration empowers introverts to make significant contributions in ways that feel authentic and fulfilling, reshaping societal perspectives on how we understand and value introversion in our rapidly evolving world.

Creating Personal Workspaces that Inspire

For introverts seeking to unlock their full potential, the sanctity of their personal workspace cannot be overstated. It's an enclave away from the frenetic energy of the outside world, a haven where ideas germinate and creativity flourishes. Crafting such a sanctuary requires both introspection and deliberate action. The goal is to foster an environment so aligned with one's spirit that it becomes a wellspring of inspiration, focus, and productivity.

One of the key principles in creating these personal workspaces is understanding what truly inspires and energizes you. Introverts often draw energy from their internal thoughts and feelings, so consider what elements in your environment evoke calm and clarity. For some, this might mean a minimalist space that reduces distractions. For others, it could involve incorporating nature-inspired elements like plants or natural light, mirroring the solace found in a quiet forest or a serene garden.

Quiet isn't just the absence of noise—it's a deliberate space for contemplation. Designing a workspace that supports this quietude is vital for introverts, who often find crowded, loud environments draining. Invest in soundproofing where possible or simply use noise-cancelling headphones to block out the hustle and bustle. These simple acts can transform a room into a sanctuary of focus and imagination.

Consider color psychology when designing your workspace. Shades of blue can evoke calmness, green inspires creativity, and earth tones offer warmth and stability. Choose colors that emotionally resonate with you and enhance your ability to work for prolonged periods without feeling fatigued. The aim is to create a visual landscape that invites rather than distracts, encouraging a seamless flow of ideas.

Beyond aesthetics, the functionality of the space should align with your daily rhythms and needs. Organize tools, resources, and furniture to facilitate efficiency. A clutter-free environment not only alleviates stress but also encourages a more methodical approach to tasks, which many introverts naturally excel in.

It's important to have a workspace that evolves with you. This flexibility is crucial for introverts, who often engage deeply and intimately with their passions. Depending on the project at hand or the current life phase, your needs might shift, demanding different stimuli or tools. Be open to rearranging or recreating your environment to reflect your current state of mind and work requirements.

Lighting, though often overlooked, plays a pivotal role in maintaining productivity and creativity for introverts. Natural light, where available, should be embraced as it promotes health and well-being, while warm, adjustable artificial lighting can fill in as necessary. This balance replicates elements of nature that rejuvenate and refresh the mind and body, essential for those who draw strength from their inner worlds.

Personal spaces should also encourage moments of reflection. Incorporate seating that's conducive to periods of rest or contemplation, allowing a break from the traditional work desk setup. Introverts often benefit from taking pauses that fuel creativity and problem-solving. A comfortable chair by the window or a quaint nook adorned with your favorite books can serve as perfect spots for reflection.

An inspiring personal workspace isn't complete without the presence of objects or art that personally resonate. Photos, quotes, or even artifacts from memorable experiences can serve as reminders of what you've achieved and what you're capable of embarking upon. They're not mere decorations but symbols of personal growth, encouragement, and the narratives of your life's journey.

While technology is a fantastic enabler of modern productivity, it's crucial to regulate its presence to prevent overstimulation or distraction, particularly for introverts, who may find excessive digital engagement draining. Create designated times for checking emails or social media to prevent these activities from encroaching on your creative flow. A balanced approach ensures that technology remains a tool rather than a deterrent.

The importance of a rejuvenating workspace extends beyond the physical domain. It's about creating a mental sanctuary, a place that echoes the introvert's identity and aspirations. This mental shift transforms the workspace from a mere location to a catalyst for achieving one's best work, bridging the gap between solitude and creativity.

In conclusion, designing a personal workspace that inspires involves a harmonious blend of select aesthetics, practical functionality, and an intentional nod to what stimulates one's senses and soul. It's about creating a symphony of elements that collectively nurture the introvert's intrinsic nature, making space for solitude to blossom into creativity and productivity. In embracing these principles, introverts can craft spaces that not only reflect who they are but also propel them towards who they wish to become.

Harnessing Solitude for Creative Growth

Solitude often conjures up images of isolation and loneliness, yet for introverts, it serves as a fertile ground for creativity and growth. In today's bustling world where constant connectivity is the norm, solitude can feel like a rare commodity. However, when deliberately chosen, moments of solitude offer a significant boost to creativity, allowing introverts to retreat into the sanctuary of their own thoughts and generate ideas with depth and originality.

Many of history's great thinkers and artists have extolled the virtues of solitude. Virginia Woolf, in her essay "A Room of One's Own," highlights the importance of having a personal space, both physically and mentally, to nurture creativity. Einstein famously pondered the universe's mysteries in solitude. These individuals were not merely escaping from the world; they were diving into their internal landscapes where creativity dwells.

For introverts, solitude is not an exile but rather an intentional retreat. It's the canvas where thoughts can be woven into new concepts without the interruptions of external stimuli. In this space of calm, introverts are free to explore their internal dialogues, letting their minds wander to unexpected places. This exploration often leads to the kind of creative breakthroughs that happen not through conscious planning but rather through a spontaneous amalgamation of thoughts.

The connection between solitude and creativity has its basis in our neurobiology. Introverts are naturally more inward-focused, with neural pathways that promote deep thinking and introspection. During times of solitude, the brain's default mode network becomes active, allowing individuals to make connections and find patterns that might not be apparent in a more crowded, bustling environment. This cognitive state facilitates the generation of novel ideas and solutions.

The act of harnessing solitude requires intentionality. It's about setting aside time where distractions are minimized, and the mind has the freedom to roam. Many introverts find creative inspiration in environments that offer tranquility—be it a serene garden, a quiet room, or the gentle hum of a library. Others may find solace in the sounds of nature, like birds chirping or waves lapping against the shore, which can act as a subtle background symphony to their creative processes.

However, it's essential to acknowledge that solitude is a double-edged sword. While it can blossom into creativity, too much solitude can lead to a feeling of disconnection from the world. The balance lies in oscillating between solitude and engagement, taking regular breaks from one's own company to recharge and reconnect with others. This balance ensures that the creative output nurtured in solitude is shared, adding value to both the creator and the community.

The power of solitude also extends to problem-solving. When introverts step away from immediate concerns, allowing their minds to settle, they discover insights and solutions that might have eluded them in crowded settings. This process isn't about forcing solutions but letting them emerge naturally. Often, the most complex problems find solutions when the mind is in a state of relaxed awareness, much like pieces of a puzzle fitting together on their own.

In workplaces that champion extroverted qualities, such as open-plan offices and constant collaboration, the value of solitude may be misunderstood. For an introvert, harnessing solitude at work might mean finding a quiet corner, using headphones to signal a do-not-disturb status, or even scheduling solo brainstorming sessions. Organizations that recognize the diverse needs of their employees can create environments that respect and incorporate the necessity of solitude for creative endeavors.

Moreover, solitude is not about doing nothing. It's an active state of being where thoughts are given room to ferment and mature. Introverts can use solitude to pursue creative hobbies—like writing, painting, or playing music—activities that offer a channel for expressing the inner world on their own terms. These creative pursuits not only fuel personal fulfillment but can also lead to innovative contributions in various fields.

Embracing solitude for creative growth also requires overcoming societal perceptions that equate aloneness with loneliness. Introverts often hear unsolicited advice to 'get out more' or 'be more social,' implying that social engagement is a benchmark for happiness and success. Yet, as highlighted by countless successful introverts, solitude can be a crucial component of personal and professional growth. It's a state where ideas can germinate without the distractions of conventional social settings.

As we continue to navigate a world that often prioritizes extroversion, the necessity of solitude for creativity must be celebrated. By understanding and embracing this powerful tool, introverts can unlock their creative potential and contribute significantly to their fields. The journey of harnessing solitude for creative growth reinforces the message that there's profound strength in quiet reflection, a reminder that some of the most groundbreaking ideas are born not from loud brainstorming sessions but from the stillness within.

Ultimately, solitude equips introverts with a unique creative palette. The ability to find clarity in silence, to explore the intricacies of their minds without external interference, is a gift. As society evolves, the narrative around solitude can shift, recognizing it as a valuable phase in the creative process rather than an indulgence.

In conclusion, when introverts embrace solitude as a space for creative exploration, they aren't just nurturing their individual potential—they're pushing the boundaries of what's possible. Solitude, with its calm and contemplative nature, offers introverts an expansive universe to explore, where ideas are not just incubated but given the freedom to soar. Through this embrace, the world can witness the vibrant tapestry of innovation and creativity introverts carry within them.

Chapter 10: Networking in an Extroverted World

In an extrovert-dominated environment, networking can feel like an uphill climb for those of us who thrive in solitude. Yet, it's entirely possible to build meaningful professional connections without abandoning our authentic selves. The strength of introverts lies in our ability to listen deeply and connect one-on-one, allowing us to forge networks that are rich in substance rather than surface chatter. It's not about becoming someone we're not, but about enhancing our natural capabilities in nuanced ways. Leveraging online spaces can serve as a great equalizer, providing platforms where we can thoughtfully engage and make our contributions felt. By embracing calculated small steps and selectively involving ourselves in aspects of networking that align with our values, introverts can craft a network that's both genuine and beneficial. The goal isn't to overwhelm ourselves but to craft connections that nurture our strengths, offering a powerful counter-narrative to the hustle-and-bustle approach typical of the extroverted world. Through self-awareness and strategic engagement, we can expand our influence while remaining true to our introverted nature.

Building Professional Networks Quietly

In a world that often equates networking with large, bustling events and enthusiastic self-promotion, introverts face unique challenges. Many networking environments are designed to cater to extroverted individuals, who thrive in social situations and gain energy from interacting with large groups. Yet, introverts possess a quiet power that can be utilized to build robust and meaningful professional networks.

Introverts, by their nature, often prefer depth over breadth. This preference is a strategic advantage in networking, allowing introverts to forge genuine and lasting connections. Instead of a scattered web of shallow contacts, introverts excel at nurturing a handful of significant relationships. In professional settings, that can translate into a network built on trust and mutual respect. The key is to recognize that networking doesn't have to mean attending every event or collecting a mountain of business cards. It can be as simple as having meaningful conversations and following up thoughtfully.

Understanding and utilizing one's natural propensity for deep listening is another facet of effective introverted networking. Introverts tend to be great listeners and observers, picking up on the subtle cues that others might overlook. This skill makes them exceptional at understanding the needs and motivations of others. By listening actively, introverts can make others feel valued and understood, often leaving a lasting impression without saying much at all.

Furthermore, the digital age has ushered in new opportunities for introverts to network on their own terms. Online platforms offer a less intimidating space where connections can be built gradually and with less pressure. Engaging in professional forums, participating in webinars, or even initiating thoughtful dialogues on LinkedIn can all serve as powerful networking strategies. These virtual interactions provide the chance to connect with others who share similar interests and goals, fostering relationships that can be just as impactful as those formed face-to-face.

Networking quietly also involves being selective about the environments one chooses to engage with. Introverts thrive in settings that allow for meaningful conversation, such as small group gatherings or one-on-one meetings. Seeking out these types of occasions can help introverts shine, as they can utilize their strengths to build connections that matter. It's about choosing quality over quantity, and recognizing that meaningful interactions can occur in quieter settings.

Moreover, introverts are typically introspective, a trait that can be leveraged when networking. By understanding their own strengths, values, and what they bring to the table, introverts can articulate their worth and interests in ways that feel authentic and comfortable. This self-awareness allows for more genuine exchanges, making the networking process more enjoyable and less draining.

Introverts can also benefit from aligning with mentors and allies who appreciate and advocate for their strengths. An effective strategy is to identify individuals in their industry who possess a complementary style or who have successfully navigated similar networking paths. These mentors can provide guidance and support, helping introverts to expand their professional circles without compromising their nature.

Networking doesn't have to be an overwhelming task. By focusing on building genuine relationships, utilizing digital platforms smartly, and choosing appropriate networking settings, introverts can quietly yet effectively expand their professional networks. The process might be different from traditional methods, but it's no less powerful. In fact, building professional networks quietly often results in connections that are deeper, more meaningful, and longer-lasting.

In this chapter of embracing our quiet strengths, it's key to remember that networking isn't about impersonating extroversion. It's about harnessing the unique advantages that introversion offers. And while extroverted methods are more visible, the quieter, more introspective approach employed by introverts can carve out equally successful professional paths. In this way, introverts can not only survive but thrive in an extroverted world, crafting a network that's both meaningful and impactful.

Utilizing Social Media as an Introvert

In a world that's increasingly digital, leveraging social media can feel like a double-edged sword for introverts. On one hand, these platforms offer a unique opportunity to connect without the immediate pressures of face-to-face interactions. On the other, the sheer volume and pace of information can be overwhelming. Yet, for introverts, social media can serve as a tool for meaningful networking and self-expression, precisely when harnessed with intention and care.

For introverts, the key to successfully navigating social media lies in deliberate engagement. Rather than spreading attention thin across multiple platforms, it's beneficial to focus on one or two that resonate the most with personal interests and comfort levels. Whether it's Twitter, Instagram, or LinkedIn, each platform has its own culture and pace. By selecting spaces that align with your strengths—be it storytelling, visual content, or professional networking—you can create a more authentic and manageable social media presence.

The beauty of social media lies in its capacity to allow introverts to express themselves on their own terms. Introverts often excel in writing and long-form content, making blog posts, thoughtful comments, and curated content sharing an effective way to engage. Rather than feeling compelled to share every detail of their lives, introverts can focus on crafting messages that are meaningful not just to others but also to themselves. This intrinsic motivation can help in building genuine connections and credibility in one's area of interest.

Moreover, introverts can take advantage of social media's boundary-setting features. Unlike in-person networking, where leaving a conversation can be socially challenging, social media allows users to regulate their engagement levels. Introverts can choose when to log on, engage, and participate in dialogues, offering them the valuable space they need to recharge. It's not about how often you're online, but how meaningful your interactions are when you are.

Using social media as an introvert isn't just about personal expression; it's also about learning and absorbing information in a way that's tailored to your pace. Curating a feed filled with content that inspires, educates, and resonates personally can turn social media into a wellspring of ideas that foster growth and learning. From following thought leaders to joining niche groups, introverts can gather insights and expand their understanding without the noise and distraction often associated with these platforms.

Another advantage of social media is the ability to connect with professionals and communities worldwide. For those who may shy away from traditional networking events, platforms like LinkedIn offer a rich ground for building professional relationships from the comfort of one's own space. Introverts can thoughtfully reach out to industry experts, join groups, and participate in discussions that elevate their personal brand and professional presence.

However, it's important for introverts to protect their boundaries while online. Engaging with social media doesn't necessitate sacrificing privacy or personal well-being. By being selective about what and when you share, and who you follow or engage with, you maintain control over your digital environment. Prioritizing quality over quantity in your interactions ensures that social media becomes a tool that works for you.

Of course, introverts should also not shy away from utilizing social media for personal enjoyment. From following art accounts to joining book clubs, these platforms can be a treasure trove of creativity and community. Discovering spaces that align with personal hobbies or passions can lead to forming connections based on genuine shared interests, thus fostering a sense of belonging without the pressure of constant interaction.

Lastly, it's crucial to remember that you're not alone in your journey. Many introverts have successfully transformed social media into a powerhouse for networking and growth. By observing how other introverts navigate these waters, you can pick up tips and strategies that could be adapted to fit your style. Whether it's setting aside specific times to engage or using scheduling tools to manage your posts, there's a multitude of strategies to explore.

In conclusion, while social media might initially seem daunting for introverts, it presents a powerful avenue to connect, learn, and express in a world where face-to-face interactions aren't always feasible. By taking a selective and purposeful approach, introverts can harness social media's potential while staying true to themselves. It's about finding the balance that enables you to engage with the world on terms that celebrate rather than overshadow the unique strengths of an introverted personality.

Chapter 11: Managing Stress and Overstimulation

In a world bustling with relentless noise and activity, introverts often find themselves overwhelmed by the flood of stimuli that can lead to stress and burnout. To navigate this, it's essential to embrace strategies that draw on introverts' natural strengths. Carving out moments of solitude for reflection and recharging is crucial—it offers the space to replenish energy and regain focus. Techniques like mindfulness and deep breathing can help maintain calmness, providing a sanctuary amidst daily chaos. Identifying personal triggers and establishing boundaries further ensures protection against overstimulation. With awareness and deliberate practice, introverts can transform potential stressors into opportunities for growth, nurturing a life that honors their quiet strengths while managing the demands of the world around them.

Techniques for Recharging and Relaxation

In a world that's constantly bustling and driven by ceaseless communication, introverts often require intentional strategies for recharging and relaxation. These are not mere indulgences but necessities for maintaining well-being and balance. The key lies in recognizing what specifically contributes to an optimal recharge process for introverts. This journey towards restoration is deeply personal, yet it resonates with common threads that many introverts can relate to.

One powerful technique for recharging is embracing solitude. Solitude doesn't equate to loneliness but rather serves as a sacred space where introverts can delve into their thoughts and feelings without the pressure to conform to external demands. It's during these quiet moments that introverts can process their experiences, recharge their emotional batteries, and emerge with renewed vigor. Setting aside time daily or weekly to be alone can offer introverts a consistent opportunity to find peace in the stillness.

Mindful practices such as meditation and deep breathing exercises offer a way for introverts to connect with their inner selves. These practices provide not only relaxation but also a heightened sense of awareness. Meditation, whether it lasts a few minutes or extends into a longer session, allows the mind to settle and creates a mental space for clarity. Deep breathing, a simple yet remarkably effective tool, can be used anywhere, from a crowded office to a serene home setting, assisting in slowing down a racing mind and diminishing stress levels.

For many introverts, nature serves as a profound and nurturing escape. Taking walks in the park, hiking through a forest, or simply sitting quietly by a body of water can foster a sense of connection to the world outside while also nurturing the inner self. Nature's rhythms have a way of centering the mind and soothing the spirit, helping introverts to recharge by offering a break from the chaotic rhythm of modern life. These natural encounters can be spontaneous or pre-planned retreats that introverts can look forward to.

Creative pursuits are another valuable avenue for introverts seeking relaxation. Activities such as writing, painting, or playing a musical instrument allow them to express themselves without the constraints of social interaction. In this space, they can lose themselves in the flow of creativity, which provides a dual benefit of relaxation and rejuvenation. These activities not only serve as a retreat but also enrich life with moments of beauty and accomplishment.

A consistent benefit for introverts looking to relax is the art of reading. Books offer a safe space for retreat and exploration, where introverts can immerse themselves in new worlds or gather wisdom from the experience of others. The beauty of reading lies in its ability to offer profound insights while simultaneously giving introverts the quietude they crave. Whether it's a novel, non-fiction, or poetry, reading is a reminder of the internal landscapes that lie within each person.

Engaging in movement, such as yoga or tai chi, blends physical activity with mental relaxation, offering a holistic approach to recharging. These practices are especially suited to introverts as they emphasize mindfulness and introspection. The slow, deliberate movements help in grounding anxiety and create a rhythmic balance between mind and body. Regular practice can build resilience against overstimulation from the outside world, providing a sanctuary of peace and vitality.

Introverts also benefit greatly from meaningful engagement with loved ones, but it's essential that these interactions respect their need for depth and sincerity. Small, intimate gatherings with people who understand and value their introverted nature can be immensely restorative. These relationships don't drain energy but instead fortify introverts, offering a support system where they can be truly themselves without fear of judgment.

Establishing boundaries is a proactive technique that supports relaxation and prevents burnout. Introverts thrive when they can delineate their limits with regard to social interactions and commitments. By clearly identifying when to say "no" and when to protect personal time, introverts can safeguard their energy reserves. This boundary-setting empowers them to engage with the world on their own terms, ensuring that they don't overextend themselves and can maintain a harmonious balance.

Finally, embracing hobbies that align with personal interests can be a rewarding way to recharge. Be it gardening, photography, knitting, or any other solitary pastime, these activities allow for focused engagement and enjoyment. Hobbies provide a constructive diversion from everyday stressors, offering an opportunity to cultivate skills and derive fulfillment from personal progress.

In summary, the techniques for recharging and relaxation discussed here reflect the unique ways in which introverts interact with the world and themselves. It's about creating a tapestry of practices that offer comfort, stimulation, and a sense of wholeness. Each technique, whether rooted in nature, mindfulness, creativity, or social connection, is a step towards nurturing the introverted self. By embracing these methods, introverts can manage stress and overstimulation effectively, finding joy and resilience in the quietude of their own company.

Recognizing and Avoiding Introvert Burnout

Recognizing introvert burnout can be a bit like trying to catch smoke with your hands—elusive but not impossible. Often cloaked in subtlety, this form of burnout doesn't explode in a dramatic outburst but rather seeps in quietly, a slow accumulation of overstimulation and emotional exhaustion. For introverts, who navigate a world often tailored to extroverted preferences, burnout can manifest through irritability, increased need for solitude, and a sense of detachment from both work and personal interactions.

Introvert burnout stems from the demand to constantly engage in environments that drain rather than recharge. Introverts are not averse to social situations; they merely manage energy differently. Stimulating environments that necessitate prolonged interaction can become overwhelming. This is akin to activating a sensory overload switch, leaving little room for recovery. The challenge lies not just in recognizing these signs early but also in knowing how to effectively recharge.

Understanding the unique triggers that lead to introvert burnout is essential in circumventing its debilitating effects. This requires introverts to become attuned to their own thresholds of stimulation. One practical strategy is to maintain a journal, documenting instances of energy drain and the circumstances that precipitate them. Over time, patterns will emerge, allowing for proactive measures and preventative planning. Identifying these triggers equips introverts with the knowledge needed to navigate an extroverted world without compromising their well-being.

Imagine a battery that drains faster than it charges. Without consistent practices to replenish, that battery soon becomes ineffective. Introverts function similarly with their energy reserves—the constant barrage of stimuli and interactions wears down their resources. Therefore, incorporating regular practices that focus on relaxation and solitude is paramount for preservation. Meditation, reading, or simply taking a walk in nature serves as an oasis in recharging one's mental energy.

Communicating one's needs is integral to avoiding burnout. This can often feel challenging in an environment that champions constant interaction and social engagement. Still, articulating personal needs for downtime or solitude to colleagues and friends serves not as a sign of weakness but as a statement of self-awareness. Encouraging others to understand and respect these boundaries fosters an environment where introverts can thrive without constant retreat.

Boundary-setting isn't just about limiting exposure to high-stimulus situations. It's about crafting a lifestyle that honors personal rhythms and respects individual capacities. Introverts can benefit from crafting tangible boundaries around work and social schedules. Scheduling regular solitude periods or quiet time is not a luxury but a necessity. Introverts should consider these boundaries as protective measures—like a well-built dam ensuring a river doesn't flood.

To mitigate potential burnout, introverts can adopt strategies that incorporate small, consistent acts of self-care. Simple practices like focused breathing exercises during brief breaks can do wonders for restoring calmness and focus. Dedicate certain times during the day free from digital distractions, allowing for moments of true stillness and reflection. This helps reconnect with one's internal landscape, maintaining equilibrium.

It is equally crucial to cultivate environments at home and work that align with introverted preferences. This doesn't necessitate major changes but involves subtle adjustments, like maintaining a clutter-free workspace, playing ambient music instead of loud tunes, or utilizing noise-canceling headphones. Creating a supportive physical environment where recharging can naturally occur facilitates a resilient shield against burnout.

Let's not forget the importance of community—creating circles of support with like-minded individuals who understand the introverted experience. Engaging in communities that prioritize similar values can significantly bolster emotional well-being and provide safe spaces to share experiences and strategies. These networks act as sanctuaries where introversion is not just accepted but celebrated as a unique strength.

In battling burnout, embracing one's introverted nature is a potent strategy. By acknowledging and valuing introverted attributes, one can begin to harness them as strengths rather than viewing them as impediments in an extroverted world. This mindset shift can be profound. Recognizing that it is permissible to decline invitations when energy reserves are low reinforces the notion that self-care is not selfish, but essential.

Finally, introverts need to remind themselves that balancing social expectations with personal needs is a dynamic process. It's about adapting and learning from each experience. Reflecting on what works and what doesn't provides the opportunity to adjust strategies effectively. Armed with this self-awareness, introverts can rewrite the narrative from defensively avoiding burnout to actively cultivating an existence that harmonizes personal authenticity with external demands.

Chapter 12: The Introvert's Guide to Social Events

Stepping into the colorful swirl of social events might feel like diving into an ocean of conversations and clinking glasses. While it can seem daunting, there's a quiet art to navigating these gatherings with grace and authenticity. Introverts needn't abandon their comfort zones entirely; instead, they can embrace their unique strengths to thrive in social settings. By setting intentional goals beforehand, such as engaging in meaningful interactions rather than numerous surface-level exchanges, introverts can transform potentially overwhelming situations into opportunities for genuine connection. Balancing social engagements with periods of solitude is crucial for maintaining energy and well-being. Recognizing personal limits and devising strategies to recharge, such as identifying quiet zones or scheduling downtime before and after events, allows introverts to participate more comfortably. Understanding that there's no one-size-fits-all approach to these experiences, introverts can empower themselves by creating their own narrative in social settings, gradually shifting both their self-perception and societal views on introversion.

Thriving in Social Gatherings

Social gatherings can be a daunting prospect for introverts, not because they lack social skills, but because these interactions often drain them of energy. Unlike extroverts who gain energy from being around others, introverts find that their mental reserves are quickly depleted in the hustle and bustle of social settings. Yet, it's entirely possible for introverts not just to survive but thrive in these situations. With the right strategies and mindset, social gatherings can become an opportunity for growth, connection, and even enjoyment.

To begin with, one of the key strategies for thriving in social gatherings lies in preparation. Introverts can benefit from setting clear intentions before attending any event. This could include determining what they hope to achieve, be it networking, learning, or simply enjoying themselves. Having a clear intention offers a sense of direction and purpose, providing a mental framework to navigate the complexities of social interactions.

It's also crucial for introverts to be selective about the events they choose to attend. Just because there's a social event doesn't mean it's essential to be there. Decide which events align with personal and professional goals, and which offer the most promise for meaningful interactions. It's better to attend fewer events with a sense of genuine interest than to spread oneself thin across many.

Once at the event, introverts often find it helpful to start with smaller, more manageable interactions. Rather than attempting to engage with the loudest or largest groups, seeking out other individuals who are alone or in smaller clusters can be more inviting. This approach not only reduces the pressure but also enhances the quality of conversations, often leading to deeper and more rewarding connections.

Remember, it's perfectly acceptable to take breaks. Social energy is limited and recognizing when to step away is crucial for maintaining comfort and stamina. Short, intentional breaks to recharge can make the difference between an overwhelmingly exhausting experience and a fulfilling one. Whether it's a quick retreat to a quieter area or a few moments of fresh air, these breaks are just as important to the overall experience as the interactions themselves.

Additionally, mastering the art of active listening can be a powerful tool for introverts. By focusing intently on what others are saying, introverts can maintain engagement without constantly feeling pressure to talk. This not only alleviates the social burden but also can lead to being perceived as more empathetic and connected, qualities that naturally align with introverted strengths.

Body language and non-verbal cues are another area where introverts can shine. Making eye contact, nodding, and offering an open posture can communicate warmth and attentiveness, allowing introverts to express interest and curiosity without needing to dominate the conversation verbally.

Leveraging technology can also enhance the social experience for introverts. Engaging with event hashtags on social media or participating in accompanying virtual components can provide a sense of involvement without the physical demands of constant in-person interaction. These methods can offer a balance, allowing introverts to connect on their terms while extending the reach of their presence.

The art of storytelling is a useful skill for introverts looking to leave a memorable impression at social gatherings. Sharing a relevant anecdote, even if brief, can passively create a deeper connection during interactions. Storytelling allows introverts to express themselves in a structured manner, focused less on improvisation and more on conveying relatable, engaging narratives.

When the event wraps up, it's vital for introverts to reflect on the experience. Analyzing what went well and what could be improved helps build perseverance and confidence for future gatherings. Think about the positive interactions, the interesting people met, and the new ideas or perspectives gained from the experience. Reflective practice encourages continuous growth and adaptability in social settings.

Incorporating these strategies, introverts can redefine their approach to social gatherings, turning them into fulfilling and enriching experiences. The realization that social success does not mean changing who you are but rather embracing your natural tendencies to connect in meaningful ways can transform the narrative around introversion in social contexts. Let's not forget introversion's unique strengths—like empathy, depth, and thoughtfulness—can leave as powerful an impact as extroverted charisma, if not more.

In summary, thriving in social gatherings as an introvert involves preparation, intentionality, and a willingness to leverage intrinsic strengths. By focusing on quality over quantity, introverts can craft a personal approach that aligns with their core values and preferences. This not only empowers introverts to participate more fully in social environments but also reaffirms the value they contribute to these spaces. Understanding these dynamics can aid in shifting broader societal perspectives, highlighting introverts as equally capable and influential participants in any social milieu.

Creating a Balance Between Socializing and Solitude

In a world that often seems geared towards extroversion, introverts can find it challenging to navigate social scenes. We're led to believe that being social is inherently good, while seeking solitude is something to be overcome. But this binary view doesn't hold water. For introverts, creating a balance between socializing and solitude isn't just a preference —it's a necessity. It's about managing energy and finding harmony in environments that may otherwise feel overwhelming. Socializing can enrich our lives, but solitude nourishes our souls.

Many introverts might feel torn between external expectations and their internal need for solitude. This tug-of-war isn't merely a social dilemma; it's a dance with our inherent nature. It's important to acknowledge that seeking solitude isn't antisocial, nor is it an escape from reality. Instead, it serves as a recharge, a necessary pause that offers clarity and renewal. Just as extroverts draw vitality from bustling environments, introverts rejuvenate through solitude. An introvert at peace with their solitude is poised and empowered in social scenarios.

Navigating social gatherings requires strategic planning. One approach is to set boundaries ahead of time. Define what the social expectations are and determine your comfort zone. The idea isn't to avoid social events entirely but to approach them with a sense of control. Maybe it means attending a party for a short duration or finding a quiet corner when things get too loud. By knowing your limits and preparing accordingly, you can maintain your energy levels without sacrificing social ties.

Furthermore, choosing the right kind of social activities can make a significant difference. Not all social scenarios are created equal. Introverts might find smaller gatherings or one-on-one meetups more fulfilling than large parties. These settings often allow for deeper connections, which align better with an introvert's preference for meaningful interactions. Imagine an evening spent with one or two close friends, sharing thoughts on life's intricacies, rather than struggling to keep up with multiple conversations at a noisy event.

Another tactic is to pair social activities with solitary pursuits. This balance can be crucial for introverts who may otherwise become drained. If you spend an afternoon at a social event, plan a few hours of quiet time for the evening. This practice doesn't just recharge your internal battery; it helps solidify the positive experiences gained from social engagement. By alternating between these states, you can fully appreciate the benefits each brings.

Perhaps one of the most empowering steps an introvert can take is to communicate their needs openly. Society doesn't always encourage expressing a desire for solitude, but advocating for your preferences can have profound impacts. Share with friends and family that solitude is how you function best, that it equips you for richer interactions. This transparency not only fosters understanding but also strengthens relationships by eliminating misunderstandings.

Additionally, mastering the art of saying "no" is essential. In an age of constant invitations and expectations to be socially active, declining offers that disrupt your balance is not only acceptable but healthy. Saying "no" isn't a refusal of others; it's a commitment to yourself. When you honor your comfort zones, you preserve the quality over the quantity of your interactions. This, in turn, maintains your well-being and enhances the interactions you choose to engage in.

Reflecting on your experiences can also be a powerful tool in creating balance. After social outings, take a moment to assess what felt right and what didn't. Was there a specific interaction that resonated? Was there anything that drained your energy more than expected? Use these insights to inform future social decisions. Self-awareness serves not as a limitation but as a guide to navigating social landscapes effectively.

Lastly, embracing one's introversion is crucial. It's about recognizing that seeking solitude isn't an obstacle to overcome but a characteristic to celebrate. Through solitude, creativity blossoms, self-discovery deepens, and resilience fortifies. When introverts accept this, they can present their authentic selves in social scenarios, bringing genuine enthusiasm rather than obligation.

Creating a balance between socializing and solitude empowers introverts to harness their full potential. It transcends a simple lifestyle choice—it's a deliberate engagement with the world that respects inner needs and enriches interpersonal connections. Rewriting the narrative around introversion also challenges societal norms, fostering environments where introverts can thrive. As we appreciate solitude not as isolation but as a form of preparation for social engagement, we embody a harmonious union between two seemingly opposing forces.

In this balance lies a profound freedom. It's the liberty to embrace our uniqueness and to orchestrate a life that aligns with our true selves. So, let's redefine the dialogue around solitude and socializing. By doing so, we can create a world where introverts not only find balance but celebrate it as a source of strength and joy.

Chapter 13: Introversion in Education

As we step into the world of education, it's crucial to recognize that introversion isn't just a personality trait—it's a different way of engaging with learning. Introverted students often thrive in environments where they can reflect and process information internally, yet traditional classroom settings can sometimes overshadow their strengths. Providing support for introverted students means crafting teaching methods that value depth over breadth, fostering spaces where quiet thought leads to profound understanding. Simple strategies like allowing for individual reflection before group discussions or offering written responses can unlock hidden potentials, transforming silence into a powerful tool for learning. Educators can play a pivotal role in highlighting and nurturing the unique abilities of introverted learners, ensuring that their quiet contributions are heard and valued. By doing so, the educational system not only empowers these students but also enriches the collective classroom experience, celebrating diverse approaches to knowledge and insight.

Supporting Introverted Students

In today's educational landscapes, introverted students often find themselves navigating environments that predominantly celebrate extroverted behaviors and learning styles. While group activities and participatory learning are vital, they're not always conducive to every student's success. It's crucial to create educational spaces where introverted students can thrive and feel valued for their unique perspectives.

Understanding introversion in an educational context begins with recognizing that different doesn't mean deficient. Introverted students often engage in deep processing; they contemplate and reflect before responding. This characteristic can lead to profound insights and innovative ideas. Educators should not only acknowledge this but also create opportunities for slower-paced, thoughtful engagement. Simple adjustments, such as providing time for reflection before answering questions or allowing written responses, can make a tremendous difference.

Moreover, classroom environments that prioritize listening as a learning tool enable introverted students to excel. Encouraging attentive listening helps in crafting a more inclusive environment. For instance, interactive lectures that invite students to jot down their thoughts can facilitate silent participation, thereby granting introverted learners room to engage at their own pace without the pressure of immediate verbal response.

Not every introverted student is shy, but many often prefer one-on-one interactions or small group settings to large, boisterous classrooms. Facilitating these kinds of interactions can help introverts build confidence and participate more actively. Instructors can design activities that pair introverts with like-minded peers, fostering a sense of security that encourages the sharing of ideas.

Providing alternative modes of participation is another essential strategy. While some students shine in oral presentations, others might produce their best work through written assignments, video projects, or creative arts. By offering multiple avenues for demonstration of knowledge, educators acknowledge diverse strengths and give all students a chance to express themselves authentically.

Additionally, teachers can cultivate a classroom culture that values alone time and solitude. It's in these quiet moments that introverts can recharge and unlock their creativity. Schools that recognize the importance of spaces for solitude (such as dedicated reading nooks or quiet gardens) provide a sanctuary for introspective rejuvenation. Encouraging students to take solo time when needed can enhance focus and mental health.

The role of educators extends beyond the classroom. They can serve as advocates for introverted students by educating peers and colleagues about the strengths of introversion. For instance, a collaborative project with the school counselor or psychologist to provide faculty training on introversion can raise awareness and promote inclusivity in the school's culture.

Schools that actively involve parents in understanding and supporting their introverted children often create a more holistic support system. Workshops and informational sessions can illuminate introverted traits and needs, providing parents with valuable tools to support their child's educational journey.

At the systemic level, policies and curriculums should evolve to recognize the diversity of learning styles. This includes rethinking standardized testing approaches and reassessing how participation and engagement are measured. Proposals for change might involve integrating reflection journals or portfolios capturing a broader range of student understanding.

Finally, extracurricular activities designed with introverted students in mind can be influential. Book clubs, art workshops, and science clubs are just a few examples of activities that let introverts shine without the overwhelming buzz of the usual extrovert-friendly options like debate clubs or sports teams. Encouraging involvement in these quieter activities can foster confidence and help introverted students expand their social circles in a comfortable setting.

A school's commitment to fostering an inclusive environment is pivotal to empowering introverted students. It involves more than just superficial acknowledgments of different personality types. Instead, it's about a deep, empathetic understanding and a willingness to adapt teaching methods to better align with varied learning needs. When structured thoughtfully, educational settings can not only accommodate but celebrate the quiet power of introverted individuals, paving the way for a future where all types of voices are heard and appreciated.

Teaching Methods that Enhance Introverted Learning

In the world of education, the needs of introverted learners have often been overshadowed by the more visible preferences of their extroverted peers. Yet, introverted students possess a unique set of strengths that, when nurtured, can lead to remarkable achievements. Educators have a golden opportunity to tap into these assets by tailoring teaching methods that enhance the introverted learning experience. This approach not only empowers introverted students but also enriches the educational environment as a whole.

Introverted learners tend to excel in settings where they can process information deeply. Reflective by nature, they prefer to tackle problems thoroughly before speaking up. This means teaching strategies that align with this preference can make a significant difference. One effective method is incorporating more written exercises and individual projects into the curriculum. These allow introverts to showcase their strengths—critical thinking, creativity, and attention to detail—without the pressure of immediate verbal responses.

Creating a classroom environment that values and promotes quiet reflection is another way to enhance learning for introverted students. While group activities have their place, offering periods of silent or independent study can give introverts the space they need to process and absorb information. This also benefits extroverted students by teaching them the value of introspection and independent work. By normalizing periods of quiet reflection, educators send a powerful message: different learning styles are respected and valued.

Teachers can also encourage introverted learning by fostering meaningful one-on-one interactions. In these settings, introverted students often feel more comfortable expressing their ideas and questions. Such interactions can be achieved through scheduled student-teacher meetings or by providing feedback via written comments. This personalized attention not only boosts the confidence of introverts but also strengthens their connection to the subject matter.

Moreover, technology offers valuable tools for enhancing introverted learning. Online discussion boards and digital collaboration platforms provide spaces where introverted students can express themselves more freely than they might in face-to-face settings. They can take the time to formulate their thoughts and contribute insights without the immediate pressure of in-person discussions. These tools enable introverts to participate actively and demonstrate their understanding in a format that plays to their strengths.

Another method involves incorporating mindfulness and relaxation techniques into classroom routines. Many introverts experience overstimulation in traditional teaching settings, with sensory inputs like noise and constant interaction draining their energy. Mindfulness exercises, such as guided meditation or simple breathing techniques, can calm the mind and increase focus. Introducing these practices not only aids introverts in managing their energy but also equips all students with lifelong skills for stress management.

It's also essential to consider the layout of the classroom itself. Establishing quieter zones where students can go to focus or reflect can be invaluable. These zones offer a retreat for introverts where they can work independently or in small groups, reducing anxiety associated with large, bustling environments. Flexible seating arrangements can further accommodate different learning preferences, allowing students to choose spaces where they feel most comfortable.

Incorporating storytelling and journaling into the curriculum taps into the introvert's affinity for exploration through writing and narrative. These techniques allow students to express their thoughts and emotions in a structured way, fostering a deeper connection to learning materials. Through storytelling, introverts can create, hypothesize, and share ideas at their own pace.

Peer-to-peer mentoring is another effective strategy that enhances introverted learning. It pairs students together in ways that promote understanding and communication. Introverts often thrive in relationships built on trust and mutual respect, and peer mentoring can create these bonds. It provides a safe space for introverts to share insights and gain confidence outside of the traditional classroom hierarchy.

Importantly, teachers should be trained to recognize and appreciate the subtler signs of engagement that introverted students display. While extroverts might dominate classroom discussions, introverts may show their enthusiasm through attentive listening and nuanced contributions. Educators who prioritize understanding these signals can better assess the true engagement levels of their entire class.

Ultimately, it's about creating an inclusive learning environment that supports diverse ways of thinking and interacting. This approach inspires confidence in introverted students, encouraging them to harness their innate talents and view their introversion as a strength rather than a hurdle. When teaching methods are adapted to embrace the quiet power of introversion, the educational landscape becomes more equitable and transformative for all students.

Chapter 14: Parenting Introverted Children

Parenting introverted children offers a unique opportunity to nurture and empower a distinct form of creativity and insight. Recognizing that introversion is not a weakness but a different way of engaging with the world can transform the parent-child relationship into one of mutual respect and growth. It's about giving them the space to retreat and recharge while ensuring they feel seen and valued for who they truly are. Understanding their quiet reflections and encouraging them to express thoughts in their own time can lead to incredible blossoming. The key is to create a supportive environment that allows introverted children to thrive, fostering their natural strengths without forcing them into extroverted molds. In doing so, parents can unlock the full potential of their children's minds, allowing their unique voices to shine brightly in a society often dominated by the loudest among us.

Encouraging Introverted Children to Thrive

Raising children is a journey filled with joys, challenges, and countless teaching moments. When you have an introverted child, the path may look a bit different, but it doesn't need to be daunting. In a world that often favors extroverted traits such as gregariousness and assertiveness, it's crucial to recognize and nurture the unique qualities of introverted youngsters. These children possess a deep well of creativity, empathy, and thoughtfulness that, when encouraged, can flourish into something remarkable.

One of the first steps in encouraging an introverted child to thrive is understanding their need for solitude. Unlike their extroverted counterparts who find energy in social interaction, introverted children often recharge by spending time alone. This doesn't mean they don't enjoy company; they simply have a different way of processing the world. Providing a peaceful and comfortable space where they can retreat allows them the freedom to relax and rejuvenate.

Acknowledging this need can be as simple as designating a "quiet zone" in the home, free from interruptions and noise. Such spaces can become havens of creativity, where children can engage fully in activities that align with their interests. Whether it's drawing, reading, or solving puzzles, these solo activities can contribute significantly to their sense of happiness and fulfillment.

Another powerful way to support introverted children is by encouraging them to express themselves through alternative forms of communication. Not every child finds words easy, especially in the heat of social interactions. Introverts might prefer writing, art, or even music as outlets for their thoughts and emotions. Parents can nurture these talents by providing the tools and encouragement needed for personal exploration and self-expression.

Listening plays an essential role in understanding introverted children. They may not always vocalize what they're feeling, but through keen observation and attentive listening, parents can gain valuable insights. Asking open-ended questions, allowing them the time to formulate responses, and respecting their opinions without interruption fosters an environment where introverted children feel safe to express themselves.

While fostering self-expression is vital, it is equally important to gently challenge introverted kids to step outside their comfort zones. Small, manageable steps can introduce them to new experiences and develop their confidence. Whether it's participating in a group project, joining a club that piques their interest, or engaging in a hobby that involves others, these experiences can help them grow socially without overwhelming their natural inclination for solitude.

Socialization, when approached thoughtfully, can be enriched by guiding them towards environments where they can interact with like-minded peers. Introverted children often form deep connections with those who share their passions and interests. Identifying and facilitating such opportunities not only supports their social development but also instills a sense of belonging.

It's vital to celebrate and highlight the strengths of introverted children. Their ability to think deeply, notice details others might overlook, and show empathy are significant assets. Reinforcing these traits cultivates positive self-perception and empowers them to value their unique contributions. Appreciation from parents and mentors can bolster an introverted child's self-esteem, reinforcing that their intuitive, thoughtful nature is powerful.

Parents can also serve as advocates for their introverted children in educational settings. By communicating with teachers and other educational professionals about their child's needs, preferences, and learning styles, parents ensure their children receive the guidance and support necessary to excel academically. Educators informed about a child's introversion are better equipped to use teaching methods that cater to diverse learning styles.

Instilling resilience in introverted children equips them to face a world that might not always understand them. Teaching them problem-solving skills, encouraging them to set personal goals, and helping them navigate challenges builds a foundation for independence. These tools prepare introverted kids to handle pressure and setbacks with grace.

Ultimately, creating an environment where introverted children feel respected and understood allows them to thrive. This involves balancing support for their natural preferences with opportunities to experience growth through positive challenges. When introverts are nurtured in a way that honors their intrinsic nature, they blossom into individuals who lead with quiet strength and authenticity.

Parenting introverted children presents a unique opportunity to cultivate the world changers of tomorrow. By prioritizing their needs, recognizing their strengths, and supporting their personal and social development, parents empower their introverted children to contribute richly to their communities and the world. As they thrive, they become living testaments to the quiet power of introversion.

Understanding and Respecting Their Needs

Parenting introverted children can feel like walking a path not often treaded in parenting guidebooks. Introverted children are often observers of the world, preferring quiet reflection over energetic exploration. Understanding and respecting the unique needs of these children is crucial to helping them thrive in environments that might otherwise overwhelm them. It's not just about accepting their nature; it's also about celebrating it and providing the right support that allows their introverted qualities to shine.

At the core of understanding introverted children is recognizing their need for solitude. Unlike extroverted kids who gain energy from social engagements and vibrant interactions, introverted children find solace and energy in being alone. This isn't a sign of antisocial behavior, but rather a critical component of their well-being. When respected, this need for solitude allows them to process their thoughts deeply, leading to a rich inner world and often, a creative mind.

Parents and caregivers can nurture this aspect by creating safe spaces for introverted children to retreat. Simple changes like designating a quiet corner in the house or scheduling downtime into their daily routines can make a world of difference. These spaces serve as a sanctuary where they feel rejuvenated and safe to express themselves without the pressures of external expectations.

However, respecting their need for solitude doesn't mean isolating them from the world. Introverted children, much like their extroverted peers, benefit from meaningful social interactions. The difference lies in the type and duration of these interactions. Smaller, more intimate gatherings with close friends or family where they can connect deeply, tend to be more fulfilling. Encouraging activities that allow one-on-one interactions, such as playing a board game or reading together, can foster these connections without overwhelming their senses.

Another key point in parenting introverted children is to be conscious of their reaction to stimuli. Loud noises, crowded places, and rapid changes can sometimes overwhelm them. Understanding this can help parents make informed choices for their children's activities. Celebrations, like birthday parties, might be more enjoyable if they are small or if the child has a quiet retreat to visit if things get too intense. It's about balancing their external activities and internal peace.

Recognizing the build-up to overstimulation is critical. Introverted children often do not vocalize their discomfort, so it's vital for parents to learn their cues—withdrawn behavior, fatigue, or irritability might signal that it's time for a break. By observing and respecting these signals, parents can prevent burnout and ensure their child remains engaged and happy.

An essential aspect of respecting their needs is advocating for them in environments that favor extroversion, such as schools. Often, educational systems prize group activities and verbal participation, which may not align with an introvert's preferred way of learning. Parents can play a role by communicating with teachers to ensure that their child's lack of vocal participation is understood and not mistaken for disinterest or disengagement. Alternative forms of participation, like written reports or small group interactions, might better showcase an introverted child's understanding and engagement.

It's also helpful to teach introverted children to advocate for themselves as they grow. Empowering them with language to express their needs—such as requesting a break or a quieter space—can build their confidence. Over time, this self-advocacy becomes a tool they can use in various situations, helping them manage their energy and interactions effectively.

Aside from understanding and advocacy, validating their experiences is profoundly impactful. Introverted children, especially in a world that often values extroverted qualities, can feel misunderstood or marginalized. Letting them know that their way of experiencing the world is valid and cherished fosters a sense of self-worth. This might involve affirming their need to spend an afternoon reading instead of visiting a busy park or sharing stories of successful introverts who have embraced their quiet nature.

Encouraging a growth mindset can also promote resilience. Introverts aren't just born; they develop and can flourish in their unique ways. Emphasizing growth allows introverted children to see challenges as opportunities rather than obstacles. They can learn to see shyness as an avenue to build courage or consider a social invitation as a chance to explore their comfort zones safely.

Finally, respecting introverted children's needs involves patience and empathy from parents. Introverted kids often require more time to open up and share their inner thoughts. Parents who exercise patience, offering their presence without pressure, create an environment where introverted children feel secure in expressing themselves at their own pace.

In conclusion, understanding and respecting the needs of introverted children isn't just crucial—it's transformative. By creating supportive environments, offering validation and advocacy, and encouraging their unique ways of connecting with the world, parents can truly empower their introverted children to grow into confident, self-aware individuals. It's a journey that requires insight and empathy, but the reward is a profound connection with a child who sees, feels, and understands the world in beautifully intricate ways. And that's worth every effort.

Chapter 15: Changing the Narrative on Introversion

As we step into the realm of changing perceptions, it becomes evident that introversion is no longer a trait to be simply tolerated but celebrated for its unique contributions to society. At the heart of this shift is the realization that diversity in personality types enriches our collective human experience. Too long overshadowed by louder counterparts, introverts bring depth, reflection, and creativity that are essential to balanced dialogue and innovation. By challenging stale stereotypes and outdated portrayals, a new narrative emerges—one that values thoughtful engagement, quiet determination, and the profound impact of subtle leadership. This transformation calls for both a media reevaluation and a societal embrace, paving the way for introverts to confidently step into their power, without feeling the need to conform or hide their true selves. It's an invitation for all to foster an environment where quiet voices are heard, and introspective minds are appreciated, catalyzing a cultural shift towards inclusivity and understanding. Through this journey, we affirm that introversion is not a limitation but a powerful attribute, reshaping how we view success and contribution.

Media Portrayal of Introverts

For decades, the media has painted introverts in a light that often doesn't reflect their true nature. From television shows to movies, the quiet and reserved characters are frequently depicted as lonely, socially awkward, or withdrawn. This portrayal, while sometimes done for comedic effect, can have profound impacts on societal perception. People start believing that introverts lack the skills needed for success, not realizing that it's this very misapprehension that masks their true strengths.

Consider the archetypal "nerd" in countless series and films. These characters are often the butt of the joke—the ones who are excluded from social gatherings or who fumble through interactions. Yet, beneath the surface of these caricatures lies a complex reality. Introverts bring unique insights, a deep sense of empathy, and the ability to listen and observe before acting. Unfortunately, media narratives usually overlook these capabilities, instead focusing on the immediate, louder interactions of their extroverted counterparts.

It's easy to understand why these portrayals resonate. Media thrives on drama and conflict, and an introvert's natural predisposition toward introspection doesn't lend itself to explosive storylines. However, the slow build of tension, the understated triumphs, and the subtle transformations that introverts often undergo can be just as compelling, if not more so. Stories of introverts lend themselves to a nuanced portrayal—a transformation within rather than an external clash.

Thankfully, shifts are occurring. We're beginning to see more rounded characters who break free from typical molds. Shows like "The Big Bang Theory" provide glimpses of introverts who, despite their awkwardness, are celebrated for their intellect and loyalty. Yet, even here, there's a delicate balance between reinforcing stereotypes and challenging them. How do we rewrite the narrative without abandoning the traits that make introverts who they are?

This doesn't mean that introverts should be shielded from criticism or challenges. Rather, it's about representing their experiences with authenticity and depth. It's about showing that the hero's journey of an introvert isn't less valid or exciting than that of an extrovert. Through more inclusive storytelling, society can embrace the diversity of thought and character that introverts bring to the table.

The book and media industry are gradually embracing this shift. Authors and filmmakers are crafting stories where introverted characters aren't just side notes but central protagonists charting their course. These characters articulate the unspoken struggles and victories of countless introverts who navigate a world skewed toward extroversion. By giving these characters a voice, art becomes a powerful tool for empathy, allowing audiences to connect deeply with the emotions and thoughts of introverts.

It's not simply about representation; it's about empowering introverts by seeing themselves reflected in the media they consume. When introverts see narratives that echo their lived experiences, it not only validates their feelings but also encourages them to leverage their unique qualities. This shift is crucial in inspiring introverts to take pride in their identity and demonstrate that there's no one-size-fits-all approach to success and fulfillment.

While significant progress has been made, there's still a long way to go in breaking the mold. The ultimate challenge is to create stories that don't just shoehorn introverts into existing frameworks but rather expand those frameworks. This means moving beyond token gestures and embracing a true understanding of introversion's many forms and intricacies.

As we move forward in this journey, media has the potential to be a powerful ally in changing the narrative on introversion. By championing authentic stories, media can help dismantle long-standing stereotypes and foster a greater appreciation for the quiet power within. Together, we can shape a cultural shift that recognizes introverts—not as anomalies, but as an integral part of the human tapestry, whose contributions are crucial and whose voices are worth celebrating.

Shifting Societal Perceptions

The tide is slowly turning, but the journey of reshaping how society views introversion is ongoing. For far too long, introversion has been misunderstood, unfairly linked with traits like shyness or even aloofness. Yet, we're currently positioned at a pivotal point where awareness is expanding, and there's a growing recognition of the unique contributions introverts bring to the table.

Look around, and you'll see more conversations highlighting the quiet strengths of introverts. Influential figures, best-selling books, and media coverage have begun to unpack the rich, inner landscapes that introverts inhabit. The notion that only the loudest voice commands attention is being challenged, offering a path to understanding that strength can lie in contemplative silence. This shift matters because it opens doors for introverts to walk through spaces once dominated by extroverted expectations.

This changing narrative isn't just happening by accident—it's a response to a broader cultural evolution. As industries evolve and careers shift towards valuing deep work, analytical thinking, and creativity, the skills often honed in quieter environments are in higher demand. Introverts, with their propensity for thoughtful reflection and listening, find themselves increasingly recognized as crucial to innovation and progress.

Yet, old stereotypes are tenacious. The portrayal of introverts in media still often leans towards caricatures of the solitary genius or the awkward recluse. We see this not just in fictional portrayals but in everyday narratives, where there's societal pressure to conform to extroverted ideals—be it in classrooms, workplaces, or social settings. Nudging societal perceptions towards balance means addressing these lingering stereotypes head-on with empathy and understanding rather than defensiveness.

It's important to recognize that shifting perceptions isn't merely about celebrating introversion but fostering an inclusive culture that honors diverse personality types. Whether we identify as introverted, extroverted, or somewhere in between, embracing a range of communication and interaction styles enriches our personal lives and professional landscapes. It's about moving beyond rigid classifications and seeing the person behind the trait.

This shift also hinges on education—illuminating both introverted and extroverted experiences in ways that foster mutual respect and appreciation. As society becomes more aware of the unique needs and strengths of introverts, we can begin tailoring educational and professional environments. By doing so, we create settings where introverts don't just cope but thrive, contributing their best without expending unnecessary energy on pretending to be someone they're not.

Introverts themselves play a vital role in this narrative change. By sharing personal experiences and stepping into roles traditionally dominated by extroverts, they redefine the possibilities for others like them. Their stories carry significant weight, dismantling misconceptions and illustrating how embracing one's true temperament leads to authenticity and fulfillment. When introverts succeed while staying true to their nature, they provide living proof that alternative paths to success exist.

Organizations can also drive change by recognizing the strengths of a balanced team. Introverted employees often excel in roles that require attention to detail, empathy, and innovation. By creating spaces that allow all personality types to flourish, companies don't just improve employee satisfaction—they leverage a wider range of insights and solutions.

In boardrooms, classrooms, and social gatherings, the conversation is expanding. People are recognizing that true collaboration arises from bringing diverse perspectives together. While changing a long-held narrative isn't easy, progress is possible when we shift focus from fitting into existing molds to understanding the multifaceted ways people contribute.

As these societal perceptions shift, introverts are increasingly encouraged to bring their nuanced perspectives to the forefront. They speak up not because they must but because they choose to share the depth of their insights. They're learning to navigate rooms that once seemed unwelcoming, and in doing so, they're paving the way for future generations of introverts.

The momentum towards reimagining introversion's place in society may start slow, but each step taken by individuals and communities echoes profoundly. With sustained effort, this wave of change promises a future where introverts not only find acceptance but are celebrated for their unique contributions. Together, we're rewriting what it means to hear and value every voice, whether it comes from the center of the room or softly from its edges.

Chapter 16: Personal Stories of Triumph

Within the rich tapestry of personal stories, introverts across the globe illuminate paths of triumph that often go unnoticed. Take Maria, who channeled her introspective nature into writing, weaving her observations into bestselling novels. Or consider James, who, despite his reserved demeanor, became a quiet force in his tech company by spearheading innovative solutions that reshaped the industry. These stories mirror a recurring theme: introverts leveraging their innate strengths—such as deep thinking and empathy—to make substantial impacts behind the scenes. Instead of succumbing to societal pressures to be louder, these individuals teach us the power of authenticity and perseverance. Their journeys underscore that success doesn't always roar; sometimes, it whispers. And in those whispers, introverts find their triumph, reminding us to value depth over volume in a world that often equates noise with achievement.

Real-Life Experiences of Successful Introverts

In a world where extroversion is often celebrated, introverts have silently been scripting their own success stories. Behind the scenes, they harness their quiet strengths to achieve remarkable feats. These stories are a testament to the fact that introversion, far from being a hindrance, can indeed be a source of profound power.

Consider the journey of Sarah, a successful software engineer at a leading tech firm. From a young age, Sarah was always more comfortable in her own company, finding solace in books and solitary walks in nature. Introversion allowed her to hone in on her analytical skills and attention to detail, both of which played pivotal roles in her career. Rather than trying to fit into roles of high-energy meetings or open-plan offices, Sarah flourished in positions that allowed deep focus and minimal interruptions. Her story reminds us that quiet spaces are fertile ground for innovation.

Similarly, Ethan, a bestselling author, attributes his literary success to his introverted nature. Writing, after all, is a solitary pursuit. Ethan's ability to delve deeply into introspection and develop complex characters comes from years of reflection and solitude. His quiet demeanor made him an excellent listener, enabling him to capture human emotions and experiences with an authenticity that resonates with his readers. Introversion offered him the introspective lens needed to view the world in vivid detail.

Then there's Maria, a scientist whose groundbreaking research in renewable energy earned her international acclaim. Maria's career showcases how introverted strengths can lead to extraordinary public achievements. Working in labs suited her preference for solo work, allowing her to meticulously comb through data and decipher complex problems without the distractions of office chatter. Her story reinforces the idea that introverts contribute immensely to innovation and discovery in fields that rely on patience and precision.

Although introversion often gets mischaracterized as a disadvantage in arenas like customer service or sales, individuals like Raj prove otherwise. As a top sales executive, his success stems from his ability to forge genuine connections and earn clients' trust. Raj listens intently, understands client needs on a deeper level, and crafts tailored solutions, contrasting the typical high-speed pitch. By leveraging empathy and thoughtful dialogue, Raj underscores how introverted traits can redefine success in traditionally extroverted professions.

Mary, a leader in a non-profit organization, exemplifies the leadership potential of introverts. Her strategic mind and ability to listen actively allow her to build cohesive and effective teams. Mary uses her introverted qualities to foster an inclusive environment, drawing out the thoughts and ideas of her team members who also tend to be quieter. This collaboration has led to numerous community-based projects that have made a tangible impact. Introverted leadership, as her example shows, can be deeply transformational.

An example from academia comes from Dr. Li, a respected professor and mentor. Dr. Li's love for quiet study and deep focus helps him engage in groundbreaking research and connect with students in meaningful ways. By understanding his students' unique strengths, many of whom are introverts themselves, he tailors his teaching to encourage discussion and contemplation. His impact extends beyond academia, influencing educational practices that highlight the importance of understanding different personality types in learning environments.

There is also the story of Alex, an introverted entrepreneur who thrives on creating innovation through solitude. Driven by his passion for technology, Alex built a successful start-up from the ground up, spending hours in isolation to perfect his product. His business approach doesn't revolve around flashy sales tactics, but rather letting the quality and functionality of his products speak for themselves. Alex's journey affirms that introverts can excel even in the entrepreneurial sphere, which might seem dominated by extroverted personas.

Unexpectedly, introverts also find success in the arts. Tess, a world-renowned painter, utilizes the quietude of her studio to channel her thoughts into vibrant expressions on canvas. Her work speaks volumes about her introspective process, drawing viewers into the beautiful complexities of her inner world. Art, for Tess, is more than an exhibition; it's a profound communication channel that transcends verbal explanation. Through her serenity and depth, Tess reminds us of the invaluable contributions introverts make to cultural enrichment.

Lastly, consider the influential role of mental health professionals, like Dr. James, an introverted therapist celebrated for his empathetic listening and keen insights. His career highlights how introverts can parse complex narratives with patience and care, providing invaluable support to those navigating life's challenges. Dr. James' approach is marked by thoughtful reflection, creating a therapeutic space where clients feel truly heard and understood. His work is a compelling example of how introversion can enhance the caregiving professions.

These stories serve not just as personal triumphs, but as beacons illustrating how introversion, with its unique strengths, is a powerful asset across diverse fields. In each narrative, the quiet persistence of introverts breaks through barriers, transforming preconceived notions of success. It's a reminder that the world benefits when everyone is encouraged to embrace their true selves. Encouragingly, these introverts jolted us to redefine success beyond the loud spotlight and find value in an introspective glow instead.

Moving forward, let us recognize and celebrate the quiet achievers among us. As society learns to value different forms of expression and contribution, we're challenged to rethink how we define and celebrate success. Real-life experiences of successful introverts not only inspire but challenge us to foster environments where every personality type can shine. Embracing these stories of triumph transforms our understanding, allowing introverts to pave new paths for future generations, shaping a world richer in diversity and understanding.

Lessons Learned from Introverted Journeys

In a world often dominated by the loudest voices and the boldest personalities, it's easy to overlook the quieter triumphs that shape our everyday lives. Introverted journeys aren't typically punctuated by grand announcements but marked by subtle victories and moments of personal clarity. The lessons learned on these paths are invaluable—not just for introverts but for anyone aiming to understand the power of quiet persistence and introspective growth.

Take a step back and imagine an introverted child, tucked away in a corner of the library, lost in the world of books. To the untrained eye, it might seem she's simply avoiding interaction. But within those pages, she's constructing worlds, drawing connections, and quietly preparing for a future she knows she can shape. This childhood scene lays the groundwork for a critical lesson: growth doesn't always occur out loud, and sometimes, the most profound transformations happen silently.

One of the most powerful lessons from introverted journeys is the realization that solitude is not synonymous with loneliness. Introverts deserve the acknowledgment that spending time alone can foster creativity, innovation, and self-awareness. Think of the greatest ideas conceived not in crowded boardrooms but in the quiet solitude of one's thoughts. By embracing solitude, introverts learn the art of listening—both to themselves and to the world around them. This skill allows for richer, more comprehensive insights into the human experience.

Success, for many introverts, is about redefining what achievement means. An introvert's journey is not necessarily a straight climb to the top but often a winding path that touches unexpected milestones. The embrace of incremental growth and the acknowledgment of small victories play a crucial role in building confidence and self-acceptance. Each task completed, every fearful situation faced, adds another layer of strength.

Resilience is another critical takeaway from introverted journeys. While extroverted peers might draw energy from external stimulation, introverts often find themselves needing to retreat to recharge. But it's in these moments of withdrawal that resilience builds its foundation. By understanding their limits and crafting strategies to manage overstimulation, introverts turn what might be seen as a disadvantage into a strength. Learning when and how to seek solace becomes a skill that guides them through personal and professional storms.

Introverted journeys also teach the value of authenticity. In environments that often reward outgoingness, introverts learn that being true to oneself is more important than conforming to external expectations. Authenticity leads to real connections and genuine interactions that feel both fulfilling and empowering. When introverts embrace their nature, they project a confidence that isn't loud but unequivocally present.

The narrative of introversion changes when we highlight the ability to observe and listen, skills that introverts naturally possess. In a team or organizational setting, this means identifying potential conflicts before they erupt, understanding nuanced interpersonal dynamics, and providing solutions that consider all angles. The power of observation, a lesson learned time and again by introverts, often leads to innovative solutions and harmonious environments.

Let's not forget that as introverts traverse their paths, they continually teach adaptability. They're adept at finding niches where they can thrive, whether by selecting careers that align with their strengths or creating work environments that accommodate their need for focused work periods. Adaptability involves marrying one's inherent traits with the demands of the outside world, turning vulnerability into an armor of flexibility.

The stories of introverted journeys also underscore the importance of strategic networking. Introverts, by nature, might shy away from traditional networking methods, but they perfect the art of meaningful, one-on-one connections. This approach nurtures deep professional relationships that aren't just transactional but transformative. They understand the power of a well-timed email, a thoughtful follow-up, and the long-term growth such interactions can foster.

Notably, introverted journeys foster an appreciation for diverse communication styles. Being on the receiving end of misunderstanding or misinterpretation instills in introverts a sensitivity toward others' perspectives. They become advocates for those who feel unheard and work toward creating an inclusive environment that appreciates varied forms of expression.

Lastly, the journey encourages introspection without becoming self-absorbing. Constant reflection helps introverts refine their sense of purpose and direction. They learn not to confuse solitude with isolation but use reflection as a tool for continual personal growth. This reflective nature enables introverts to align their actions with their core values, creating a path that is both meaningful and fulfilling.

The lessons drawn from introverted journeys are many—and when shared, they enrich the broader tapestry of human development. By embracing the power of introspection, authenticity, and strategic solitude, introverts not only find triumph but also a unique space from which to lead and inspire others. Such lessons provide all of us with a different lens through which to view success, reminding us that there is no singular path to achievement, but a multitude of ways to make a profound impact.

Chapter 17: Introversion Across Cultures

Introversion, while sharing core traits, manifests uniquely across the world's diverse cultures, offering both a common thread and a kaleidoscope of expressions. In places where collectivism prevails, like in parts of Asia, introverted traits are often seen as virtues—emphasizing harmony, patience, and humility—while in more individualistic societies, like the United States, these same qualities might be misunderstood or undervalued. This cultural lens influences not just the perception of introversion but also provides unique opportunities for introverts to harness their strengths. From Scandinavian countries, where introspective thought is prized, to Mediterranean cultures, where vivacity is more celebrated, understanding and appreciating these cultural nuances empowers introverts to navigate their environments with greater confidence and authenticity. Embracing this diversity not only enriches our global perspective but also encourages introverts everywhere to assert their voices, knowing that introversion holds universal value and transformative potential.

Cultural Variations in Understanding Introversion

Introversion is a globally shared personality trait, yet it's interpreted differently across cultures. These variations teach us that while the essence of introversion—a preference for quieter environments and thoughtful reflection—remains consistent, cultural expectations and values shape how introversion is perceived and experienced. Understanding these differences gives us a broader perspective on what it means to be an introvert, freeing us from singular narratives and empowering us to be ourselves in diverse settings.

In many Western cultures, such as the United States, there's an emphasis on assertiveness, outgoing behavior, and individual achievement. It's often a society that celebrates extroversion, sometimes leaving introverts feeling out of place or undervalued. However, this environment also breeds resilience in introverts. They learn to navigate a landscape that doesn't always celebrate their natural temperament, fostering adaptability and strength.

By contrast, some Eastern cultures, like Japan and China, often hold introverted traits in high regard. Here, being quiet and reserved is sometimes seen as a form of respect and thoughtfulness. For instance, in Japan, silence is valued as a sign of wisdom and a way to demonstrate sincerity. Introverts in such societies might find themselves more naturally in tune with cultural expectations, allowing their reflective nature to shine without reservation.

This variance is not only seen between Eastern and Western cultures but also within regions. In Scandinavia, for example, the social demeanor can lean towards introspection and privacy, aligning well with introversion. People living in these regions might feel more comfortable seeking solitude without the societal push to constantly engage, a testament to the understanding built into their cultural fabric.

Interestingly, in cultures with a community-oriented mindset, like those in parts of Africa and Latin America, introversion can present a unique challenge. These cultures emphasize interpersonal relationships and collective participation, sometimes creating friction for introverted individuals who don't naturally gravitate toward large social gatherings. However, even here, introverts find their niches—often contributing through deep, meaningful connections rather than broad social circles.

Europe's diverse cultural landscape offers its own tapestry of understanding introversion. In Southern Europe's more vibrant and community-focused societies, introverts might need strategies to maintain their energy, while Northern European countries might offer environments more conducive to introspection. This spectrum within a relatively small geographical area underscores the profound impact culture has on the perception of personality traits.

Acknowledging these cultural variations isn't just an intellectual exercise; it's a call to action for introverts globally. Knowing where they come from, different cultures aren't just caveats in a broader discussion— they're lived realities that shape introverts in unique ways. When introverts travel or interact with cultures different from their own, this understanding promotes empathy and adaptability, allowing them to honor their true selves while respecting cultural norms.

From a global perspective, introversion is not monolithic. It reminds us that personality traits are a complex blend of intrinsic qualities and cultural feedback. As we start to appreciate the nuance of cultural variations, we encourage a more inclusive worldview. This cultural awareness doesn't just benefit introverts; it enriches everyone by promoting greater understanding and acceptance of diverse identities.

To be an introvert is to navigate a world rich in cultural complexity. By recognizing cultural differences, introverts can reframe challenges into opportunities for growth. No longer isolated by societal misconceptions, they unlock the potential to thrive globally. Embracing cultural diversity is a journey that underscores a broader mission to redefine introversion —not just locally but across the world.

The journey of understanding cultural variations in introversion ultimately reveals a more profound truth: in the tapestry of human experience, variation is strength. While cultural contexts shape the expression of introversion, the core values of introspection and authenticity remain universal. This global appreciation of introversion is not just an academic study—it's a celebration and empowerment of what it means to be truly oneself, regardless of cultural constraints.

Thus, as introverts and those invested in understanding introversion, recognizing and respecting cultural variations propels us toward a more nuanced and unified perspective. It inspires us to embrace difference, fosters empathy, and illuminates paths for introverts to flourish authentically, no matter where they are in the world. The world is vast and varied, yet these cultural nuances offer valuable lessons for everyone, reminding us to honor and cherish our unique introverted journeys worldwide.

Cross-Cultural Success Stories of Introverts

In a world that often prizes extroverted qualities, introverts might feel they have to adapt to fit an extrovert's mold. But what's truly enlightening is discovering how introverts from various cultures have not only survived in environments that might seem inhospitable to their natures but have thrived. These stories of triumph and innovation culminate in a tapestry of cross-cultural success. They remind us all that the seeds of greatness lie deep within, waiting to be cultivated in any setting. Let's explore the remarkable journeys of those introverts who, regardless of cultural expectations, have left indelible marks on their fields.

Consider the story of a renowned Japanese architect whose minimalist yet profound designs earned international acclaim. In Japan, a society that often values collectivism and harmony, introversion can be seen as both a challenge and an asset. This architect seamlessly blended introspective thought with cultural aesthetics, crafting spaces that speak the language of quietude and reflection. The result is a body of work that not only celebrates introversion but also enhances communal tranquility, showcasing how introverted strength can reshape cultural landscapes.

On the other side of the globe, a Tunisian scientist made groundbreaking strides in renewable energy. In North Africa, where community gatherings are deeply embedded in daily life, this scientist found her solace in the solitary pursuit of research. Her relentless curiosity and attention to detail carved out a niche in a field dominated by collaborative practices. By choosing to focus on individual contribution and problem-solving skills, she developed sustainable technologies that are now making waves worldwide. Her success story shatters the myth that introversion is a drawback, illustrating the power of the focused pursuit of knowledge.

In Sweden, a country noted for its appreciation of individualism, one introverted author used intimate and nuanced storytelling to address some of society's biggest challenges. Through her quiet demeanor and profound imagination, she crafted narratives that brought attention to mental health and environmental issues. Her novels inspire empathy and invite readers to reflect, demonstrating how the thoughtful articulation of ideas can influence public discourse across cultural boundaries. This introvert's ability to connect deeply with readers is a testament to the universal appeal of introspective insight.

The tech industry has often been a beacon for introverts who prefer to communicate through code rather than conversation. An Indian software developer turned her preference for deep thought and solitude into a global phenomenon by developing an innovative app that supports mental health. Her design, rooted in the cultural values of mindfulness and meditation, resonates with users around the world. This introvert's journey underscores how personal passions and quiet resilience can spark advancements that have lasting, cross-cultural impact.

Then there is the story of a Brazilian artist whose vibrant yet serene paintings have captivated art lovers far beyond her native country. Amid the energetic samba and colorful festivals that characterize much of Brazil's identity, she found her voice in the calmness of her studio. Her art, which explores themes of introspection and solitude, invites viewers to appreciate the quiet moments in life. This highlights how introverted creativity can contribute richly to cultural dialogues, offering new perspectives and experiences.

Crossing into the business realm, a German introverted entrepreneur transformed her introversion into an asset, leading her start-up to international success. In a business landscape that often encourages assertiveness and directness, she excelled through her ability to listen and empathize with both employees and customers. Her leadership style, rooted in thoughtful consideration and strategic planning, proved that the qualities of an introvert could indeed translate to the flourishing of a global enterprise.

Finally, consider the experience of a Kenyan journalist who, despite the vibrant and dynamic media environment, leveraged her introverted talents to produce poignant, in-depth investigative pieces. Her quiet determination and exceptional listening skills allowed her to uncover stories that others might have overlooked. By amplifying the voices of the marginalized, her work not only challenged societal narratives but also demonstrated the profound impact of introverted persistence in raising awareness and inspiring change.

These stories collectively underscore a powerful message: introverts can transcend cultural expectations and redefine success on their terms. Whether in art, technology, business, or any other field, the quiet resolve and unique perspectives of introverts have the potential to transform industries, enrich communities, and inspire generations. By embracing their innate strengths, introverts from every corner of the globe not only find their place but also redefine what it means to thrive in a culturally diverse world.

As we celebrate these cross-cultural successes, they remind us all of one crucial truth: the quiet flame of introversion, when nurtured, can illuminate paths previously unseen. Cultural norms may vary, but the core qualities of introversion—focus, introspection, and thoughtful innovation—are universal. Through understanding and valuing these traits, we can continue to empower introverts everywhere to share their light with the world.

Chapter 18: Introverts and Technology

In today's rapidly evolving digital landscape, introverts are finding novel opportunities to leverage technology as a powerful ally, enhancing their inherent strengths while redefining their roles in society. The digital realm, often overwhelming to some, offers introverts the gift of solitude while fostering far-reaching connections. Whether through immersive online communities or innovative productivity tools, technology empowers introverts to curate environments that build on their quiet strengths. By selectively engaging with social media and utilizing virtual platforms, introverts can participate in meaningful dialogues and collaborations without the social exhaustion that traditional settings might induce. As we delve into this digital age, it's clear that technology serves not just as a tool but as an expansive canvas, allowing introverts to express their creativity and assert their presence in ways that were previously unimaginable. This fusion of introversion and technology illuminates a path toward a future where quiet voices are amplified, not overshadowed, ensuring that introverts continue to thrive in a world that's more accommodating and inclusive than ever before.

Thriving in a Digital Age

In a world increasingly mediated by screens and devices, introverts find themselves in a paradoxical position. On one hand, the quiet confines of a digital world suit their natural inclinations for reflection, solitude, and deep thinking. On the other, the incessant buzz of notifications and the pressure to be constantly available online present new challenges to their equilibrium. Yet, this digital age offers unprecedented opportunities for introverts to shine, leveraging their unique qualities to navigate, adapt, and thrive.

The digital world offers an array of tools that introverts can harness to express themselves effectively without the immediate pressure of face-to-face interaction. For instance, the art of written communication flourishes online, providing introverts with the time and space to carefully consider their words before sharing them. This suits the innate tendency of many introverts to think twice before they speak, allowing for more thoughtful and nuanced contributions that resonate deeply with listeners and readers alike.

Social media, often seen as a realm for extroverts, offers introverts a platform to craft and control their narratives. Through blogs, forums, and social networking sites, they can connect with like-minded individuals from around the globe, forming communities that transcend physical boundaries. These digital spaces provide introverts with a considerable sense of belonging and recognition, empowering them to engage in meaningful exchanges on their terms.

However, introverts must also navigate the challenges posed by a digitally interconnected world. The allure and addiction of social media can lead to a sense of overstimulation—a state introverts typically strive to avoid. Learning to manage digital noise and setting boundaries becomes essential. By carefully curating their online environments and adopting a mindful approach to digital consumption, introverts can protect their inner peace while engaging with the wider world.

One of the most significant advantages of the digital age is the ability to work remotely. This shift offers introverts the chance to thrive in a working environment tailored to their preferences. The elimination of open-office distractions, the ability to structure the workday around personal productivity peaks, and the comfort of a personal workspace provide introverts with conditions conducive to their success.

Technology also offers dynamic ways for introverts to express creativity and innovation. Many find solace in the quiet spaces of digital creation, using tools like graphic design software, music production apps, and writing platforms to channel their creative energies. The digital age transforms introverts from passive consumers into active creators, allowing them to make significant contributions while maintaining their sense of autonomy and individuality.

Moreover, introverts can harness technology to amplify their learning and professional development. Online courses, webinars, and virtual workshops offer introverts the flexibility to read, reflect, and absorb information without the social pressures of a traditional classroom. This type of learning environment can encourage deeper engagement and more focused attention, aligning perfectly with the strengths of introverted personalities.

In embracing technology, introverts not only find ways to strengthen their skills and reach broader audiences but also gain the confidence to assert themselves more visibly in various spheres. As they become more adept in navigating the digital landscape, they can execute their ideas and insights more effectively, thereby enhancing their influence and impact.

Furthermore, digital platforms are redefining networking opportunities. For introverts, the traditional networking events could feel daunting, but virtual networking offers a much-needed reprieve. The online world allows introverts to initiate and nurture professional connections through emails, LinkedIn, and industry-specific virtual forums at their pace, granting them the confidence to build a robust network without physical constraints.

Nevertheless, with great power comes great responsibility. The digital age demands a level of digital literacy and savvy that ensures introverts don't get overwhelmed by the pace and scale of online interactions. Introverts are encouraged to develop digital consciousness—an awareness of how online behaviors affect their psychological well-being. By adopting mindful technology use, they can maintain the balance necessary for personal and professional fulfillment.

Ultimately, thriving in a digital age as an introvert involves embracing technology as a tool for growth while staying true to one's nature. This era may indeed redefine the parameters of success for introverts, emphasizing quality over quantity, and genuine connections over fleeting interactions. As introverts take charge of their digital domains, they naturally reshape societal perspectives, proving that their voices are not just relevant but essential in the dialogue of our time.

Using Technology to Enhance Introverted Strengths

In a world that's become increasingly digital, technology offers introverts a unique opportunity to leverage their natural strengths. Gone are the days when the loudest voice in the room automatically commanded the most attention. Today, different forms of technology empower introverts to express their ideas, connect with like-minded individuals, and thrive through means that align with their innate preferences and talents.

One of the most compelling benefits of technology for introverts is the ability to communicate thoughtfully. Email, messaging apps, and social media platforms allow for introspective contemplation before responding—something that face-to-face interactions don't always permit. When introverts communicate online, they can tap into their strengths of reflection and deep thinking. This leads to interactions that are not only thoughtful but deeply insightful.

Also, many introverts find the ability to review and edit their written communications comforting. Online, they can take the time to express themselves without the pressure of immediate response. This careful approach can enhance communication by allowing for more meaningful exchanges—a boon for anyone who thrives on well-articulated thoughts rather than spontaneous banter.

Moreover, technology has revolutionized the ways in which introverts can network. Unlike the bustling and often overwhelming environments of traditional networking events, online forums and professional networks like LinkedIn provide introverts with the chance to connect on their terms. These platforms enable one-to-one communications, allowing introverts to form deep, meaningful professional relationships without the social anxiety that might accompany in-person events.

Another area where technology can augment introverted strengths is in the realm of remote work. The emergence of digital workspaces means that many introverts can work in environments where they feel most comfortable and productive. Remote work allows introverts to minimize unnecessary social interactions and create workspaces that inspire creativity and productivity. This flexibility not only boosts efficiency but also improves job satisfaction and mental well-being.

With the surge in digital tools, technology also provides introverts with new avenues for lifelong learning, an area where they naturally excel. Online courses, webinars, and virtual workshops offer introverts the room for independent study—one of their core strengths. These platforms empower them to delve into subjects of interest and develop skills without the immediate pressures of a physical classroom or the fast-paced interactions that might dominate traditional learning environments.

Social media is another technological facet that introverts can use to enhance their strengths. While social networks might seem to cater to extroverted personalities, introverts can use these platforms strategically. By carefully curating their social feeds and engaging selectively, introverts can cultivate a digital environment that reflects their interests and passions. This tailored approach can not only keep introverts informed and inspired but also connect them with communities that share their values and beliefs.

For introverts who are artistically inclined, digital media and online platforms offer unparalleled opportunities to showcase their creative talents to a global audience. Introverts often possess rich inner worlds brimming with creativity. Technology gives them the tools to transform these internal ideas into tangible creations. From blogging to podcasting to publishing e-books, introverts can share their unique perspectives with the world without stepping into the spotlight in traditional ways.

Furthermore, technology's role in facilitating deeper understanding can't be overstated. Virtual reality and immersive technologies can provide introverts with incredible experiences that were previously unavailable. These tools offer introverts new ways to engage with content, explore different perspectives, and deepen their understanding of the world—all without the social overstimulation that might accompany real-world experiences.

Looking at mental health, which is a significant concern for introverts, technology offers apps and online resources dedicated to mindfulness and mental well-being. These can be incredibly beneficial for introverts seeking to manage stress or requiring time to recharge. Apps offering guided meditations, calming music, and stress management techniques can create a safe mental space for introverts, helping them cultivate inner peace in a chaotic world.

Employers have started recognizing the potential that digital tools hold for introverts. In the workplace, introverts can utilize project management tools, collaboration platforms, and internal social networks to contribute effectively without feeling the need to be constantly vocal. By fostering an environment that embraces digital communication, employers can create a more inclusive workspace where introverts feel valued and can showcase their strengths.

Technology, in essence, unshackles introverts from the confines of traditional interaction patterns. It provides a stage where their voices can be heard in the most authentic and impactful ways possible. Introverts are poised to redefine how success is measured in our increasingly digital world. By aligning external demands with their internal states, introverts can carve out a fulfilling and impactful niche.

Therefore, it's crucial for introverts to stay attuned to technological advancements. The ever-evolving digital landscape holds opportunities waiting to be explored. By embracing these digital tools and adapting to change, introverts will not only enhance their natural strengths but also inspire others who share those quieter, yet powerful, inclinations.

In the digital age, understanding how technology can augment their strengths can open doorways introverts might not have previously imagined possible. Whether it's enhancing communication, boosting creativity, or facilitating connections, technology is an ally to the introvert —ever ready to assist them in expressing their true selves and turning their quiet power into something vibrantly influential.

Chapter 19: The Future of Introversion

In a world that increasingly values diverse perspectives, the future of introversion holds exciting possibilities. As society evolves, more people recognize introversion not as a quirk to be altered but as a unique lens through which profound insights and innovations arise. Advances in technology and shifts in workplace dynamics are setting the stage for environments where quiet contemplation and thoughtful consideration, traits intrinsic to introverts, are not merely accepted but celebrated. As these trends gain momentum, introverts can find confidence in navigating spaces that once seemed solely the domain of the extroverted. There's an empowering movement forming—a collective awakening to the idea that introversion is not a barrier, but a strength. By embracing these changes, introverts are not only preparing to thrive but also to lead in ways that resonate with authenticity and depth, shaping the narrative of tomorrow with their rich, inner worlds.

Emerging Trends Affecting Introverts

The world is rapidly transforming, driven by technological advancements, shifting societal norms, and global connectivity. These changes are introducing new scenarios and challenges that particularly resonate with introverts. As we move forward, introverts will find both opportunities and obstacles woven into the fabric of these emerging trends, requiring them to adapt while staying true to their nature.

Remote work is a trend that has gained significant traction, partly accelerated by global events such as the pandemic. This shift can greatly benefit introverts by providing the solitude they cherish, along with the flexibility to structure their workday around their energy cycles. Introverts often perform better in environments where they can minimize interruptions, and working remotely provides a buffer against the often crowded and bustling settings of traditional offices.

However, a fully remote work environment isn't without its challenges. Introverts may face difficulties in establishing genuine connections with colleagues through screens alone. The lack of face-to-face interactions can lead to a sense of isolation, potentially impacting professional relationships and collaboration. To counteract this, introverts might need to consciously engage in virtual social activities or opt for hybrid models that offer occasional office interactions.

Another significant trend is the increasing importance of soft skills in professional settings. The dynamics of leadership and teamwork are evolving, with a greater emphasis on empathy, active listening, and emotional intelligence. These skills align well with introverted tendencies, as introverts typically excel at one-on-one interactions and reflective thinking. For introverts, capitalizing on their inherent soft skills can open new doors and foster career development.

Yet, mastering these skills in larger groups remains a nuanced challenge. Introverts may feel the pressure to emulate extroverted behaviors, particularly in environments that favor overt enthusiasm and constant engagement. Balancing authenticity with adaptation becomes crucial, as introverts strive to showcase their strengths without compromising their comfort.

The digital age continues to evolve with social media platforms gaining unprecedented influence. For introverts, this presents both opportunities and drawbacks. The ability to craft thoughtful responses and engage in deep, meaningful conversations online can be empowering. Social media allows introverts to connect with like-minded individuals globally, expanding their community without the conventional demands of face-to-face interactions.

On the downside, the constant barrage of notifications and the expectation to always be "on" can be overwhelming. Introverts may sometimes feel pressured to participate in discussions or digital networking, which can lead to digital fatigue. Finding a balance between engagement and setting personal boundaries will be key to thriving in this new landscape.

Moreover, as technology proliferates, the emergence of artificial intelligence and virtual realities are reshaping everyday experiences. These tools promise to revolutionize how introverts learn, socialize, and even entertain themselves. Virtual reality can simulate environments where introverts can practice social interactions without the immediate pressure of real-world scenarios. However, reliance on these digital realities comes with the risk of alienation from tangible, in-person experiences.

Introverts might also engage with AI-driven platforms that offer personalized content attuned to their preferences. While this can enhance productivity and enjoyment of technology, it's essential to be mindful of the echo chambers that algorithms can create, inadvertently limiting exposure to diverse perspectives and ideas.

In broader societal shifts, there is a growing acknowledgment of mental health and well-being, with introversion increasingly being recognized as a natural personality type rather than a disadvantage to overcome. This trend encourages environments that are more inclusive of diverse personality types, supporting introverts in expressing themselves authentically. The advocacy for mental health in workplaces and educational institutions bears the potential to reduce stigma around introversion and create spaces where introverts feel welcomed and supported.

Despite these positive changes, introverts may occasionally encounter environments resistant to transformation. Traditional expectations linger in various industries and social circles, where extroversion is often seen as the default trait for success. Advocating for introvert inclusivity in such settings requires ongoing effort—paving the way for acceptance through awareness and education.

In navigating these evolving trends, introverts have the opportunity to redefine success on their own terms. By harnessing their innate strengths—such as their ability to focus deeply, think critically, and communicate thoughtfully—they can excel across various fields, leading to a more expansive understanding of leadership and achievement. As introverts carve new paths, they contribute to reshaping cultural narratives, gradually shifting the perception of introversion from a quiet quirk to a powerful asset.

Looking ahead, it's crucial for introverts to continue advocating for their needs and preferences, ensuring that they aren't sidelined in a rapidly changing world. Engaging in networks and communities where their voices are valued can offer support and validation. There's a collective journey awaiting introverts, one where they can inspire others to embrace their own unique traits, ultimately fostering a future that's as diverse in its appreciation of personality as it is inclusive in its opportunities.

Preparing for the Future as an Introvert

In a world that's rapidly evolving, introverts stand at a unique crossroads, poised like never before to make significant contributions while working in harmony with their inherent nature. The future demands skills and qualities that introverts naturally excel at: introspection, focused attention, and a profound ability to listen and think deeply. At the heart of this preparation lies the ability of introverts to anticipate changes, adapt accordingly, and utilize their strengths to navigate uncharted territories.

As we look to the future, it's vital for introverts to prioritize self-awareness. Knowing oneself, recognizing personal strengths, and understanding areas of comfort and discomfort will serve as a foundation upon which to build other skills. The increasing emphasis on emotional intelligence and interpersonal sensitivity in personal and professional settings plays directly to an introvert's strengths. By continuing to cultivate these qualities, introverts can create resilient support structures tailored to their unique needs.

Technology offers another powerful avenue for introverts to flourish in the future. Digital platforms enable introverts to connect deeply without the pressures of face-to-face interactions. Introverts can harness these tools to create robust networks that don't drain their energy, allowing them to engage with the world on their own terms. Asynchronous communication, online collaborations, and spaces for reflection and creativity are just a few aspects where technology and introversion intertwine beautifully.

Furthermore, it's essential for introverts to prepare for an increasingly collaborative world by developing strategic communication skills. Introverts may prefer solitude and quiet, but this doesn't mean they can't thrive in teams or lead effectively. Learning to communicate their ideas compellingly, using clarity and thoughtfulness, can allow introverts to make meaningful contributions. Workshops, mentorships, and real-world practice can provide introverts with necessary tools to hone their communicative prowess.

The future workplace places an increasing value on diversity of thought, and this extends significantly to the styles and strengths of introverted individuals. Organizations are slowly but surely recognizing that a diverse team includes diverse personalities which enrich the fabric of collective creativity and innovation. Introverts who prepare themselves by participating in conversations around inclusivity, advocating for their needs, and seeking environments that align with their values will be better positioned to thrive.

Moreover, introverts can look ahead with optimism when considering the potential shifts in traditional educational and work structures. As remote working becomes more commonplace, introverts are finding environments that allow them to channel their energies towards work without unnecessary overstimulation. Similarly, digital nomadism offers an exciting opportunity—an introvert can immerse themselves in new environments at their own pace, offering a rich tapestry of cultural experiences minus the conventional constraints.

Resilience will be a key trait for introverts as they prepare for the future. Resilience is not about overcoming adversity with brute strength but rather about flexibility and adaptability—qualities that introversion nurtures. By approaching challenges with a mindset oriented towards growth and learning, introverts can turn what might seem like obstacles into stepping stones. Building resilience involves continuous learning, reaching out for support, and structuring life in ways that respect the ebbs and flows of energy that introverts experience.

Finally, as society collectively redefines success, it is crucial for introverts—and indeed, everyone—to anchor their understanding of fulfillment and achievement in personal values rather than external validation. Introverts can prepare for the future by aligning their life's trajectory with their passions and what truly matters to them. By doing so, they're more equipped to make decisions that foster personal and professional growth without compromising their well-being.

The path forward for introverts is filled with possibilities. With strategic self-awareness, an embrace of technology, an understanding of evolving paradigms of success, and an unwavering dedication to authentic living, introverts can indeed flourish in the future. They hold the key to not just adapting to a changing world but also shaping it in ways that favor depth, genuine connection, and thoughtful innovation. As the world leans into more complex challenges, the quiet power of introverts could not be more relevant or necessary. The future, after all, is shaped in the moments of quiet reflection and deliberate action where introverts naturally thrive.

Conclusion

As we embark on the journey of understanding and harnessing the power of introversion, it's essential to recognize the significance of breaking free from long-standing stereotypes. Throughout this book, we've aimed to empower introverts and shift societal perspectives. We've delved into the underlying science, celebrated introverted leaders, and explored the nuances of effective communication and career success for those who often thrive in quieter spaces.

The world needs introverts—individuals who bring depth, creativity, and thoughtfulness to their endeavors. They've historically steered profound changes and contributed richly to various fields. Recognizing this quiet strength has the potential to enrich workplaces, communities, and personal relationships.

Acceptance and self-celebration lie at the heart of embracing one's introverted nature. By acknowledging the distinct traits that make introverts who they are, individuals not only foster self-growth but also help cultivate a more inclusive society. Introverts offer an authentic perspective that values depth over superficiality, encouraging us all to take time to pause and reflect.

In personal and professional settings, introverts thrive by leveraging their inherent strengths. This involves choosing careers aligned with their natural dispositions and adopting strategic approaches to challenges like office dynamics or public speaking. It's about finding one's way to communicate and connect deeply without sacrificing personal authenticity.

It's not just about surviving in a world designed with extroverts in mind; it's about thriving and influencing change. Introverts possess unique qualities that can redefine leadership, drive innovation, and enhance creativity. As more introverts step into leadership roles, they prove that different dynamics do not equate to lesser value—rather, they often bring a refreshing balance.

Building meaningful relationships and comfortable workspaces allows introverts to express their true selves. Setting boundaries and cultivating deep connections helps them navigate the complex social fabrics of life without feeling overwhelmed. Moreover, social media and technology are powerful tools, providing introverts with platforms to engage comfortably and creatively without the constraints of traditional social settings.

Education systems and parenting approaches have a profound impact on introverts. Understanding and nurturing introverted students and children ensures their potential is not only recognized but celebrated, allowing them to flourish in their own unique ways. Education tailored to enhance their learning styles makes way for confident, self-assured individuals.

The narrative of introversion, unfortunately, has often been shaped by myths and misconceptions. By presenting real-life stories of triumph and cultural variations, we've highlighted how introversion transcends boundaries, influencing societies and cultures differently. It's a testament to the universal value introverts bring to our global tapestry.

Looking forward, trends suggest a world more accommodating to diverse personalities, where introversion isn't regarded as a hurdle but as a legitimate, powerful force. As technology evolves, introverts stand poised to harness new opportunities, ensuring they remain influential and impactful in countless sectors.

As we stand on the brink of a new understanding of introversion, let's pledge to continue advocating for and supporting the introverted individuals around us. Whether it's in personal circles or global platforms, promoting a narrative that values quiet strength is essential. Introverts have always been here, contributing silently yet substantially, and it's time the world not only acknowledges but celebrates this invaluable contribution.

This book is just the beginning. May its lessons resonate, inspire, and catalyze ongoing conversations that illuminate the quiet power within. Here's to embracing introversion and all its wonders, leading us towards a future of deeper connections and richer experiences.

Appendix A: Resources for Introverts

In the journey of embracing one's introverted nature, having the right resources can make all the difference. Whether you're seeking insightful books or digital tools to bolster personal growth, this collection offers a wealth of options designed specifically for introverts. These resources range from recommended reading that dives deep into the nuances of introversion to supportive communities and networks where introverts can feel understood and empowered. With the right guidance, introverts can harness their unique strengths, cultivate self-awareness, and connect meaningfully with others. By exploring these resources, introverts will find inspiration and practical advice to thrive in both personal and professional spheres, transforming society's understanding of what it truly means to be introverted.

Recommended Reading and Tools for Development

In our journey to embrace introversion and tap into its power, resources can serve as invaluable guides. Books, articles, and software tools can enlighten and equip us in the quest to foster personal and professional growth. They provide insights, strategies, and affirmations that can lead to a deeper understanding of oneself, especially in navigating a world that often seems to celebrate extroversion above all else.

Among the essential readings, consider diving into literature that explores the essence of introversion and its role in society. These books often provide a profound understanding of how introverts can thrive in various settings, emphasizing the strengths that come with this personality trait. Such texts stand as testimonies and guides, inspiring introverts to capitalize on their natural inclinations rather than masking them.

One standout book worth mentioning centers around the concept of quiet strength and how introverts bring subtler, yet impactful, contributions to leadership and innovation. It's a call to introspection and action, helping readers align their gifts with their career paths and life goals. Through real-life examples and well-researched narratives, it reinforces the notion that introversion is not to be overcome but embraced and celebrated.

In addition to reading material, digital tools designed to enhance personal development and productivity can be particularly effective for introverts. Apps that facilitate mood tracking, meditation, and mindfulness practices can help manage stress and encourage moments of solitude that restore energy. By integrating these tools into daily routines, introverts can create a personalized balance that nurtures both their mental health and productivity.

Furthermore, leveraging platforms that foster professional development can be a game-changer. Online learning communities and courses offer an avenue to gain new skills and knowledge without the hustle and bustle of traditional settings that may overwhelm introverted individuals. Such environments allow for self-paced learning and introspective absorption of material, aligning perfectly with introverted learning styles.

It's also beneficial to engage with writers and thinkers who dedicate their work to exploring introversion in various cultural and societal contexts. Their research and insights can broaden one's perspective on how introversion is perceived globally, revealing both universal and unique aspects that can influence personal strategies for growth and adaptation.

Journaling is another tool that facilitates introspection and personal growth. Keeping a journal can help introverts process their thoughts and feelings more effectively. It's a safe space to reflect on experiences, set goals, and track progress. This practice can be a quiet yet powerful way to nourish personal development and self-awareness.

On the technological front, software that simplifies task management and enhances productivity can be invaluable. Tools with features like customized workspaces and reminders allow introverts to work uninterrupted, building environments aligned with their need for focus and reduced social interaction. These digital assistants ensure that tasks and projects are organized and executed efficiently, contributing to a sense of achievement and reducing stress.

Connecting with others through virtual platforms can also be instrumental. Online communities where introverts share resources, experiences, and encouragement foster a sense of belonging and collective growth. These networks are crucial for introverts seeking companionship and solidarity without needing constant physical interaction.

In summary, the pursuit of personal and professional development for introverts is well-supported by a wealth of resources. By engaging with thoughtfully curated readings, supplementing them with practical tools, and drawing wisdom from a global perspective on introversion, introverts can unlock their full potential. These resources serve to empower, offering a roadmap for navigating life's challenges while embracing the unique strengths inherent in introversion.

Supportive Communities and Networks for Introverts

In a world that often feels dominated by extroverted ideals, finding spaces where introverts can thrive becomes essential. For introverts, the need for supportive communities and networks can't be overstated. These spaces offer solace, empowerment, and understanding, forming a foundation where introverts are celebrated for who they are rather than pushed to change. The growth of online platforms and networks has opened up a myriad of opportunities for introverts to connect with others from the comfort of their homes, creating environments that value thoughtful dialogue over relentless chatter.

Online communities have emerged as powerful tools for introverts seeking connection. Platforms such as forums, social media groups, and niche online communities provide a space to share experiences and insights. These environments respect personal space and pace, allowing introverts to engage on their own terms. Through these virtual networks, introverts can exchange advice, support, and encouragement. Whether it's discussing strategies for self-care, sharing personal achievements, or tackling challenges unique to introverts, these spaces serve as a collective brain trust of introverted knowledge.

Beyond digital realms, local meetups and gatherings tailored for introverts have become increasingly popular. Quiet clubs and minimalist events curate experiences designed specifically to accommodate the introvert's need for low-stimulus environments. These gatherings emphasize the quality of interaction rather than quantity, making it easier for introverts to engage deeply without feeling overwhelmed. By attending small, focused group events, introverts can form meaningful connections that align with their natural social rhythms.

Book clubs, writing groups, and hobbyist circles also offer excellent avenues for introverts to connect with like-minded individuals. These groups naturally allow for introspection and deep conversation, making them ideal for those who prefer engaging in shared interests over small talk. Introverts benefit by immersing themselves in activities that bring joy and fulfillment while simultaneously building a support network. Such communities often become lifelines where introverts can recharge and grow, fostering a sense of belonging that's both enriching and comforting.

Professional networks specifically aimed at introverts are gaining momentum as well. Many professionals find networking daunting, especially when traditional methods center around high-energy events. Introvert-friendly networking groups focus on creating spaces where introverts can excel, emphasizing authentic relationships over transactional interactions. These networks encourage genuine conversations that tap into the unique strengths of introverts, such as empathy, active listening, and detail-oriented thinking. As a result, introverted professionals can expand their connections and discover career opportunities without sacrificing their core identities.

In addition to formal networks, informal mentor-mentee relationships can be especially beneficial for introverts. Having a mentor who understands the nuances of introversion can be invaluable. Mentors provide guidance, share experiences, and offer pathways to greater self-awareness and career success. These relationships can often transcend professional advice, as mentors become trusted confidants who help mentees navigate both personal and professional landscapes.

Furthermore, therapeutic communities play a vital role in supporting introverts. Therapy groups and support forums tailored for introverts allow individuals to explore their temperament in a safe, validating environment. These settings help introverts process experiences of overstimulation and societal pressure, often incorporating techniques like mindfulness and stress management. Participating in such communities can lead to personal breakthroughs, as introverts learn to embrace their nature and build resilience.

One of the most critical aspects of supportive communities is the shared understanding they provide. Being among those who inherently understand the introvert's experience can alleviate feelings of isolation and self-doubt. Members of such communities frequently report feeling seen and heard in ways they hadn't experienced before. This sense of recognition not only nurtures confidence but also empowers introverts to assert their needs and boundaries in broader societal contexts.

Educational institutions and workplaces are increasingly recognizing the importance of creating inclusive environments that cater to diverse personality types. Introverts are finding more spaces where their contributions are valued, whether through quiet zones in libraries and workplaces, or through the introduction of policies that support diverse working and learning styles. Aligning with such communities can be transformative, allowing introverts to forge paths that are true to their idiosyncrasies and ambitions.

Ultimately, supportive communities and networks provide introverts with more than just a place to belong. They offer a launchpad for personal development, creativity, and empowerment. In these environments, introverts can flourish, using their quiet power to make significant impacts both in their personal lives and the wider world. As introverts build and nurture these communities, they not only support themselves but also shift societal perceptions, paving the way for a more nuanced understanding of introversion's role in our collective narrative.